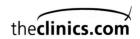

Agnes E. Rupley, DVM, Dipl. ABVP–Avian
CONSULTING EDITOR

VETERINARY CLINICS

OF NORTH AMERICA

Exotic Animal Practice

Endocrinology

GUEST EDITOR
Anthony A. Pilny, DVM, Dipl. ABVP–Avian

January 2008 • Volume 11 • Number 1

SAUNDERS

An Imprint of Elsevier, Inc.
PHILADELPHIA   LONDON   TORONTO   MONTREAL   SYDNEY   TOKYO

W.B. SAUNDERS COMPANY
A Division of Elsevier Inc.

Elsevier, Inc., 1600 John F. Kennedy Blvd., Suite 1800, Philadelphia, PA 19103-2899

http://www.vetexotic.theclinics.com

VETERINARY CLINICS OF NORTH AMERICA:	**Volume 11, Number 1**
EXOTIC ANIMAL PRACTICE	**ISSN 1094-9194**
January 2008	**ISBN-13: 978-1-4160-5835-9**
Editor: John Vassallo; j.vassallo@elsevier.com	**ISBN-10: 1-4160-5835-4**

The ideas and opinions expressed in *Veterinary Clinics of North America: Exotic Animal Practice* do not necessarily reflect those of the Publisher. The Publisher does not assume any responsibility for any injury and/or damage to persons or property arising out of or related to any use of the material contained in this periodical. The reader is advised to check the appropriate medical literature and the product information currently provided by the manufacturer of each drug to be administered to verify the dosage, the method and duration of administration, or contraindications. It is the responsibility of the treating physician or other health care professional, relying on independent experience and knowledge of the patient, to determine drug dosages and the best treatment for the patient. Mention of any product in this issue should not be construed as endorsement by the contributors, editors, or the Publisher of the product or manufacturers' claims.

Veterinary Clinics of North America: Exotic Animal Practice (ISSN 1094-9194) is published in January, May, and September by Elsevier, Inc.; Business and Editorial offices: 1600 John F. Kennedy Blvd., Suite 1800, Philadelphia, PA 19103-2899. Customer Service Office: 6277 Sea Harbor Drive, Orlando, FL 32887-4800. Subscription prices are $161.00 per year for US individuals, $288.00 per year for US institutions, $84.00 per year for US students and residents, $190.00 per year for Canadian individuals, $333.00 per year for Canadian institutions, $202.00 per year for international individuals, $333.00 per year for international institutions and $101.00 per year for Canadian and foreign students/residents. To receive student/resident rate, orders must be accompanied by name of affiliated institution, date of term, and the *signature* of program/residency coordinator on institution letterhead. Orders will be billed at individual rate until proof of status is received. Foreign air speed delivery is included in all *Clinics* subscription prices. All prices are subject to change without notice.

POSTMASTER: Send address changes to *Veterinary Clinics of North America: Exotic Animal Practice*; Elsevier Periodicals Customer Service, 6277 Sea Harbor Drive, Orlando, FL 32887-4800. **Customer Service: 1-800-654-2452 (US). From outside of the US, call 1-407-345-1000.**

Veterinary Clinics of North America: Exotic Animal Practice is covered in *Index Medicus*.

Printed in the United States of America.

CONSULTING EDITOR

AGNES E. RUPLEY, DVM, Diplomate, American Board of Veterinary Practitioners–Avian; Director and Chief Veterinarian, All Pets Medical & Laser Surgical Center, College Station, Texas

GUEST EDITOR

ANTHONY A. PILNY, DVM, Diplomate, American Board of Veterinary Practitioners–Avian; Avian and Exotic Pet Medicine, Lenox Hill Veterinarians, New York, New York

CONTRIBUTORS

SUE CHEN, DVM, Diplomate, American Board of Veterinary Practitioners–Avian; Gulf Coast Avian and Exotics, Gulf Coast Veterinary Specialists, Houston, Texas

BOBBY R. COLLINS, DVM, MS, Diplomate, American College of Laboratory Animal Medicine; Director, Division of Animal Resources, Virginia Commonwealth University, Richmond, Virginia

RICARDO DE MATOS, LMV, Diplomate, American Board of Veterinary Practitioners–Avian; Lecturer, Section of Wildlife and Exotic Medicine, Department of Clinical Sciences, College of Veterinary Medicine, Cornell University, Ithaca, New York

CHRISTINE ECKERMANN-ROSS, DVM, CVA, Associate Veterinarian, Avian and Exotic Animal Care, PA; and Adjunct Associate Professor, North Carolina State University College of Veterinary Medicine, Raleigh, North Carolina

BRAD LOCK, DVM, Diplomate, American College of Zoological Medicine; Assistant Curator of Herpetology, Department of Herpetology, Zoo Atlanta, Atlanta, Georgia

CHRISTOPH MANS, Med Vet, Avian and Exotic Animal Service, Veterinary Teaching Hospital, Ontario Veterinary College, University of Guelph, Guelph, Ontario, Canada

ANTHONY A. PILNY, DVM, Diplomate, American Board of Veterinary Practitioners–Avian; Avian and Exotic Pet Medicine, Avian and Exotic Pet Medicine at Lenox Hill Veterinarians, New York, New York

MIDGE RITCHIE, BA, Ross University School of Veterinary Medicine, Basseterre, St. Kitts, West Indies

DRURY R. REAVILL, DVM, Diplomate, American Board of Veterinary Practitioners–Avian; Diplomate, American College of Veterinary Pathologists; Citrus Heights, California

SAM RIVERA, DVM, MS, Diplomate, American Board of Veterinary Practitioners–Avian; Associate Veterinarian, Department of Animal Health, Zoo Atlanta, Atlanta, Georgia

ROBERT E. SCHMIDT, DVM, PhD, Diplomate, American College of Veterinary Pathologists; Zoo/Exotic Pathology Service, Greenview, California

ELISABETH SIMONE-FREILICHER, DVM, Diplomate, American Board of Veterinary Practitioners–Avian; Avian and Exotic Medicine Department, Veterinary Medical Center of Long Island, West Islip, New York

W. MICHAEL TAYLOR, DVM, Avian and Exotic Animal Service, Veterinary Teaching Hospital, Ontario Veterinary College, University of Guelph, Guelph, Ontario, Canada

CONTENTS

and describes the etiology, diagnosis, and treatment of diabetes mellitus in pet birds.

Adrenal Steroid Metabolism in Birds: Anatomy, Physiology, and Clinical Considerations

Ricardo de Matos

The hypothalamo-pituitary-adrenal system in birds is anatomically and functionally different from that in mammals. The adrenal gland structure and corticosteroid hormone physiology of birds will be reviewed. The anatomy and physiology sections of this article will be important for better understanding the pathogenesis, diagnosis, and possible treatment of primary or secondary adrenal gland disease. Causes of hyper- and hypoadrenocorticism in birds also will be reviewed. The article will conclude with current indications and complications to the clinical use of glucocorticoids in birds.

Calcium Metabolism in Birds

Ricardo de Matos

Calcium is one of the most important plasma constituents in mammals and birds. It provides structural strength and support (bones and eggshell) and plays vital roles in many of the biochemical reactions in the body. The control of calcium metabolism in birds is highly efficient and closely regulated in a number of tissues, primarily parathyroid gland, intestine, kidney, and bone. The hormones with the greatest involvement in calcium regulation in birds are parathyroid hormone, 1,25-dihydroxyvitamin D_3 (calcitriol), and estrogen, with calcitonin playing a minor and uncertain role. The special characteristics of calcium metabolism in birds, mainly associated with egg production, are discussed, along with common clinical disorders secondary to derangements in calcium homeostasis.

Update on Neuroendocrine Regulation and Medical Intervention of Reproduction in Birds

Christoph Mans and W. Michael Taylor

In avian species, reproductive disorders and undesirable behaviors commonly reflect abnormalities in the neuroendocrine regulation of the reproductive system. Current treatment options are often disappointing, show no long-lasting effect, or have significant side effects. A possible reason for our lack of success is a dearth of knowledge of the underlying neuroendocrine, behavioral, and autonomous physiology of the reproductive processes. Tremendous progress has been made in the last few years in our understanding of the neuroendocrine control of reproduction in birds. Advantage should be taken of these experimentally derived data to develop appropriate and safe treatment protocols for avian patients suffering from reproductive disorders.

maintained as pets, biomedical research animals, or display animals in zoos. The clinical diagnosis of endocrine diseases almost never occurs in free-ranging animals in their native habitat. Feral animals that have clinical endocrine disease, such as neoplasia, adrenal cortical hyperplasia, or diabetes, would exhibit clinical signs of altered behavior that would result in their removal by predators. The diagnosis of endocrine disease thus takes place in the relatively protective environment of captivity. This observation should forewarn pet owners and clinicians caring for these animals that the environment contributes to the development of endocrine diseases in these animals.

The field of reptilian clinical endocrinology is still in its infancy. The thyroid and parathyroid glands are intimately involved with many basic metabolic functions. These glands have been the subject of extensive research studies in reptilian species; however, the effects of abnormal gland function have been poorly documented in clinical cases. These glands play a major role in maintaining physiologic homeostasis in all vertebrates. With the advent of more sensitive assays, it should be possible to measure the small amounts of hormones found in reptilian species. The purpose of this article is to review the literature regarding clinical endocrinology of the thyroid and parathyroid glands in reptiles.

FORTHCOMING ISSUES

RECENT ISSUES

Preface

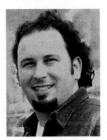

Anthony A. Pilny, DVM, DABVP–Avian
Guest Editor

For many veterinarians treating avian and exotic pets, diseases of the endocrine system make for challenging subject matter. The inclusion of an endocrine disorder on the differential diagnosis list can be intimidating and the diagnostic approach and treatment options even more daunting. A myriad of testing protocols, therapeutic options, and reference ranges are either anecdotal or extrapolated from canine and feline medicine—or simply do not exist at this time. There are few rules "carved in stone" regarding diagnosis and treatment of endocrine disease in the entire field of veterinary endocrinology and, in many cases, even less information about companion birds and exotic pets.

Another way to look at this dilemma is to simply accept that much remains to be learned. Endocrine physiology can differ greatly among species, especially when comparing veterinary to human medicine. This means the field of avian and exotic pet endocrinology offers great potential for research, investigation, case studies, protocol development, and therapeutic options for a given patient. As clinicians continue to medically work up difficult cases and apply sound medical skills, we all benefit and gain knowledge of diseases of the endocrine system.

I am privileged to be guest editor for this issue of *Veterinary Clinics of North America: Exotic Animal Practice* devoted to endocrinology. The field of endocrinology is complex and unique, and knowledge of endocrine disease is significant and thought-provoking. Although there are some well-known endocrine disorders seen in clinical practice, much is still unknown about the exact pathophysiology and subsequent treatment of these conditions. In

1094-9194/08/$ - see front matter © 2008 Elsevier Inc. All rights reserved.
doi:10.1016/j.cvex.2007.10.001

some cases we still do not even know if our patients can develop certain disorders or if current methods of diagnostic testing are useful. We are also lacking normal reference ranges for many species. My goal with this issue is to provide a mix of information, including new developments, detailed physiology, and clinically relevant material for the practitioner.

The talented contributors to this issue were asked to update the most current information on their topics and also to include anatomy, physiology, and biochemistry when relevant to broaden our understanding of the endocrine systems. This allows readers to become better informed and make rational clinical decisions when attempting to diagnose and treat endocrine disease.

I offer my sincere appreciation and gratitude to the contributors to this issue. I also thank John Vassallo for giving so much time and assistance to the publication of this issue. The topics were challenging and everyone put much time and effort into presenting an excellent review of endocrinology of avian and exotic pets.

Anthony A. Pilny, DVM, DABVP–Avian
Avian and Exotic Pet Medicine, Lenox Hill Veterinarians
204 East 76th Street, New York, NY 10021
Animal Specialty Center
9 Odell Plaza, Yonkers, NY 10701

E-mail address: apilny@avianexoticpetvet.com

ELSEVIER
SAUNDERS

VETERINARY
CLINICS
Exotic Animal Practice

Vet Clin Exot Anim 11 (2008) 1–14

The Anatomy and Physiology of the Avian Endocrine System

Midge Ritchie, BA[a],*,
Anthony A. Pilny, DVM, DABVP–Avian[b]

[a]*Ross University School of Veterinary Medicine, PO Box 334,
Basseterre, St. Kitts, West Indies*
[b]*Avian and Exotic Pet Medicine, Lenox Hill Veterinarians,
204 East 76th Street, New York, NY 10024, USA*

The avian endocrine system is comparable to that of mammals and consists of eight glands: the pituitary-hypothalamus complex, the gonads, pancreatic islets, adrenal glands, thyroid glands, parathyroid glands, ultimobranchial glands, and the endocrine cells of the gut (Fig. 1). The hormones secreted by these glands are released into the bloodstream to help regulate cellular function. Hormones are also a system of regulation that complements the nervous system, which regulates the muscular and secretory activities, whereas the endocrine system regulates metabolic function. Avian endocrinology is an area that is frequently unfamiliar to practitioners; however, it is important to have a thorough understanding of normal endocrinology because abnormalities may be more frequently diagnosed. It is of vital importance to always confirm a clinical presentation of an endocrine disorder before beginning treatment. It may be difficult to confirm a diagnosis once treatment has been started, and improper or inadequate treatment can be fatal. Specific diseases and treatments are not covered in this article—only the anatomy and physiology of normal patients. Please refer to other articles in this journal for more information on specific endocrine organ systems.

The pituitary gland

Anatomy

The pituitary gland, also known as the hypophysis, is a small gland that lies at the base of the brain and is connected to the hypothalamus. It is

---

* Corresponding author.
E-mail address: mritchie@rossvet.edu.kn (M. Ritchie).

1094-9194/08/$ - see front matter © 2008 Elsevier Inc. All rights reserved.
doi:10.1016/j.cvex.2007.09.009

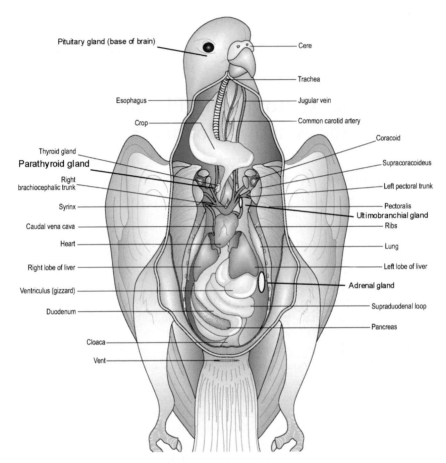

Fig. 1. Diagram of a psittacine bird shows the anatomic location of the endocrine glands. The gonads are not pictured. (*Modified from* O'Malley B. Clinical anatomy and physiology of exotic species. London: Elsevier; 2005. p. 131; with permission.)

physiologically separated into two distinct portions: the anterior pituitary (adenohypophysis) and the posterior pituitary (neurohypophysis), each of which originates from different embryologic sources. In mammals, the adenohypophysis forms the pars distalis, the pars intermedia, and the pars tuberalis. There is no pars intermedia in birds; therefore, the adenohypophysis is comprised of the pars distalis (anterior pituitary gland) [1]. The pars distalis is separated into a cephalic and a caudal lobe. The neurohypophysis is made up the pars nervosa (posterior pituitary gland), the infundibular stalk, and the median eminence. The pars distalis makes up most of the adenohypophysis and is ventrally situated to the neurohypophysis.

Six important hormones are secreted by the adenohypophysis, all of which play a major role in metabolic function throughout the body (Table 1). Two separate gonadotropins (follicle-stimulating hormone [FSH] and

Table 1
Hypothalamic releasing and inhibitory hormones

Hormone	Primary action
Luteinizing hormone–releasing hormone	Stimulates secretion of FSH and LH by gonadotropes
TRH	Stimulates secretion of TSH by throtropes, GH release by somatotropes, and prolactin by lactotropes
GHRF[a]	Stimulates secretion of growth hormone by somatotropes
Somatostatin–growth hormone inhibitory hormone	Inhibits secretion of growth hormone by somatotropes
VIP	Stimulates secretion of prolactin by lactotropes
Dopamine–prolactin-inhibiting hormone	Inhibits prolactin release by lactotropes
CRF[a]	Stimulates secretion of ACTH by corticotropes

Abbreviations: ACTH, adrenocorticotropic hormone; CRF, corticotropin-releasing factor; FSH, follicle-stimulating hormone; GHRF, growth hormone-releasing factor; TRH, thyrotropin-releasing hormone; TSH, thyroid-stimulating hormone; VIP, vasoactive intestinal peptide.

[a] As of yet, growth hormone–releasing factor and corticotropin-releasing factor have not been isolated in birds; however, studies have shown that increases in each hormone have occurred when birds were injected with mammalian homologs.

luteinizing hormone [LH]), growth hormone (GH), thryrotropin, prolactin, and adrenocorticotropic hormone (ACTH) are all secreted by the anterior pituitary gland. The neurohypophysis consists of the neurosecretory terminals, and two important hormones are released—either mesotocin or arginine vasotocin (AVT). These two hormones are secreted from separate neurosecretory neurons, and their cell bodies are located in overlapping areas within the hypothalamus. AVT and mesotocin are transported bound to carrier proteins and then stored in the pars nervosa until released.

Physiology

Adenohypophysis
Gonadotropins. Avian LH and FSH are glycoproteins that consist of two subunits, an α-subunit and a β-subunit, both of which are required for activity. LH is mainly secreted from the caudal lobe, and its major role in female birds is to stimulate ovarian steroid synthesis to induce ovulation. A surge of LH concentrations is seen 4 to 6 hours before ovulation and is low during egg laying, incubation, and care for the chicks. The concentration rises again toward the end of the chick-rearing period to prepare for the next egg-laying cycle [2]. In male birds, LH stimulates the Leydig cells to differentiate and produce testosterone, whereas FSH promotes Sertoli cell differentiation and spermatogenesis. LH and FSH are essential for controlling testicular function. Research has shown that gonadal function is regulated by daylight length. Japanese quail, when exposed to long daylight periods (8–20 hours), had an increase in testicular size and a rise in plasma

LH and FSH concentrations. Other factors, such as nutritional deficiencies and increased stress, can influence gonadotropin synthesis negatively.

The secretion of LH and FSH is under the control of luteinizing hormone–releasing hormone, although its ability to influence FSH is not completely understood. A chicken radioimmunoassay is used to measure plasma LH levels in other avian species; to measure FSH plasma concentrations, the mammalian radioimmunoassay can be used [2].

Thyrotropin. Avian thyroid-stimulating hormone (TSH) is assumed to be similar to its mammalian homolog, a heterodimer that consists of α- and β-glycoprotein subunits. TSH is produced by thyrotropes, which are cells located in the cephalic lobe of the anterior pituitary gland [3]. The main role of TSH is to stimulate avian thyroid growth. TSH also increases the release of thyroxine (T_4) from the thyroid glands. Studies have shown that injection of TSH in chickens is followed by an increase in circulating concentrations of tri-iodothyronine (T_3) and T_4. TSH does not directly increase T_3 release; rather it stimulates T_4 release, which is rapidly converted to T_3.

The release of TSH is predominately under hypothalamic control. In mammals, TSH release is under stimulatory control by thryotropin-releasing hormone (TRH). The case is similar in birds; TRH has been found in the chicken hypothalamus [1]. Other studies have shown that TRH stimulates TSH in vitro and in vivo. T_3 exerts a negative feedback effect on TSH release, as it does in mammals. It is also believed that environmental factors and dietary restrictions influence TSH release. There are no homologous radioimmunoassays for avian TSH. It has been reported that human TSH radioimmunoassay detects immunoreactive TSH in the plasma of Japanese quail [4].

Somatotropin. The somatotropes are located in the caudal lobe of the anterior pituitary gland. GH is a small protein molecule that has a molecular weight of approximately 23,000 daltons. During late embryologic development and early posthatch life, the number of somatotropes increases rapidly until a plateau is reached. Avian GH has been isolated from pituitary tissue, and the cDNA for chicken GH has been sequenced. There is evidence of variants, which seem to be caused by posttranslation modifications [5].

All the major anterior pituitary hormones exert their principal effects by stimulating target glands except for GH, which does not function through a target gland but exerts its effects directly on all or almost all tissues of the body [6]. GH is required for normal posthatching growth. It causes growth of almost all tissues of the body that are capable of growing. It is thought that GH exerts its effect on somatic growth by increasing circulating concentrations of insulin-like growth factor-I via stimulation of insulin-like growth factor-I from the liver [7].

GH has several other specific effects in addition to its effect on growth. There is evidence that GH has short-term effects on metabolism by stimulating lipolysis, exerting an insulin-like effect on inhibiting glucagon-stimulated lipolysis, and reducing lipogenesis. Other effects of GH include influencing the adrenal cortex to release corticosterone, having a stimulatory effect on the immune system, and stimulating T_4 release, although it is not formally established [1].

Release of GH from the pituitary gland is under hypothalamic control, and there are three hypophysiotropic factors in birds, two of which are stimulatory. The major stimulus for GH release is TRH, which is found to potentiate GH release factor–induced GH release in vivo and in vitro. GH release factor is thought to be another contributing factor to the release of GH, although avian GH release factor has not yet been isolated. Mammalian GH release factor has been found to increase GH release in chickens, however. The last factor, somatostatin, plays an inhibitory role in the control of GH release. It has been found that synthetic somatostatin (SRIF) depresses GH response to TRH in domestic fowl in vivo and in vitro.

Because chicken and turkey GH has been isolated, a radioimmunoassay is available for avian GH. Radioreceptor assays for avian GH have been established, and effects of physiologic state on chicken GH mRNA levels have been quantified by Northern blot analysis [8].

Lactotropin. Prolactin has been isolated and recombinant chicken prolactin has been purified after expression in *Escherichia coli*. Lactotrophs are restricted to the cephalic lobe of the pars distalis, and the proportion changes with physiologic state—it is higher in newly hatched birds than in adults [1].

Prolactin is involved in incubation behavior and can act to reduce circulating concentrations of gonadotropins. In turkeys, prolactin has proven to increase nesting activity and, with sex steroids, to induce incubating behavior. Circulating levels of prolactin are increased during incubation and fall rapidly if the behavior is interrupted. Prolactin is believed to be involved in photorefractoriness, which is the inability to respond to a stimulating photoperiod. It also stimulates the production of "crop milk" and the increase in mucosal cells of the crop sac gland in pigeon and doves, which has been used as the biologic assay for prolactin. During the last stage of incubation, the crop increases in weight and there is an increase in the plasma prolactin concentrations. It is also possible that prolactin directly influences behavior in pigeons and doves because prolactin receptors have been found in the brains of doves [9].

The major factor that stimulates prolactin release is vasoactive intestinal peptide, which has been identified in the hypothalamus. Other factors that stimulate prolactin release are TRH and AVT. Dopamine has been shown to inhibit prolactin secretion [1]. Homologous radioimmunoassays have been developed for avian prolactin. A heterologous prolactin radioimmunoassay also can be used to measure prolactin [1].

Corticotropin. Avian ACTH, similar to its mammalian homolog, is a simple polypeptide. ACTH is synthesized as part of a large protein, pro-opiomelanocortin, that contains the sequences of β-endorphin, which is part of β-lipotropin. All of these have been purified in several avian species. ACTH is produced by the acidophilic cells of the anterior pituitary gland, and it coexists in the same cells as α-melanophore–stimulating hormone [1]. ACTH stimulates the adrenal cortical cells to produce corticosterone, aldosterone, and deoxycorticosterone; its effect is mediated by cAMP [10]. The secretion of ACTH is under the control of hypothalamic-hypophysiotropic factors and glucocorticoids and presumably corticotropin-releasing factor, although it has not yet been characterized. Mammalian corticotropin-releasing factor has been shown to stimulate ACTH release in vitro from chicken and duck pituitary cells [11].

Neurohypophysis

Arginine vasotocin and mesotocin. The hormones of the neurohypophysis have been isolated: AVT, the avian antidiuretic hormone, and mesotocin, the oxytocin principle [12]. AVT is the major antidiuretic in birds. It has been shown that without it, there is a large increase in the amount of urine [13]. At low concentration, AVT exerts its chief effect of tubule function and at higher concentrations it reduces the glomerular filtration rate. Noticeable but contradictory cardiovascular effects of AVT have been reported in birds. It can have vasodepressor and vasopressor activities, depending on how it is administered [1].

Oviposition is also controlled by AVT. At the time of oviposition, circulating concentrations of AVT are greatly increased. The pars nervosa is the likely source of AVT, but ovarian AVT may contribute significantly; follicular AVT levels decline immediately before oviposition [14]. It is believed that the neurohypophyseal peptides control the secretion of other hormones; for example, AVT stimulates prolactin release in vitro and ACTH secretion [1].

Little is known about the physiologic role of mesotocin in birds; unlike its mammalian homolog, it does not seem to affect the uterus [15]. Mesotocin does, however, influence blood flow to some organs and reduce circulating concentrations of aldosterone [16].

The thyroid gland

Anatomy

The thyroid glands are paired oval glands located ventrolaterally to the trachea, caudal to the junction of the subclavian and common carotid arteries. The histology of avian thyroids is like those of mammals. It is organized into follicles filled with a secretory substance, colloid, and lined with cuboidal epithelial cells that secrete into the interior of the follicles. The major constituent of colloid is thyroglobulin, which contains the thyroid hormones within its molecules. This storage allows for a large stock of reserve thyroid hormone. Calcitonin cells, which are the chief or parafollicular cells in mammals, are absent in the avian thyroid. They are located in separate ultimobranchial organs [17].

Physiology

Although investigations of avian thyroid function are less comprehensive than those of mammals, histologic and physiologic data indicate that the mechanisms of hormone synthesis and release by avian thyroid glands are essentially the same as those in mammals [17]. As in other vertebrates, T_4 and T_3 are also the avian thyroid hormones. The first stage in the formation of thyroid hormones is the transport of iodides from the blood into the thyroid glandular cells and follicles. The rate of iodide trapping by the thyroid is influenced by several factors, the most important being the concentration of TSH. Uptake of radioiodide by the avian thyroid is rapid and retention time is prolonged. Both of these factors are influenced by dietary iodide availability [17].

The thyroid gland is unusual among the endocrine glands because it has the ability to store large amounts of hormone. Thyroid hormones are stored in the follicular colloid and formed within the thyroglobulin molecule. Thyroglobulin itself is not released into the circulating blood in measurable amounts; instead, T_4 and T_3 are first cleaved from the thyroglobulin molecule and then the free hormones are released. In adult birds with adequate iodide intake, the thyroids contain primarily T_4, with almost undetectable amounts T_3. T_4 concentrations greatly exceed those of T_3 in avian plasma. This relationship is much less extreme than in the thyroid gland itself [18]. Adult birds have plasma or serum T_4 concentrations in the range of 5 to 15 ng T_4/mL and T_3 concentrations in the range of 0.5 to 4 ng T_3/mL. Plasma and serum concentrations of both hormones have been measured in many avian species [18].

Upon entering the blood, the thyroid hormones combine immediately to plasma proteins. The major transport proteins in birds are albumin and prealbumin/transthyretin [17]. Binding proteins serve several functions: they maintain an extrathyroidal hormonal store, they maintain tissue hormone supply if thyroid gland function varies, and they are a factor in the regulation of hormone supply to the tissues. Transthyretin also may play a more specific T_4 supply role by transporting T_4 through the choroid plexus into the brain [19].

The avian thyroid gland is primarily under the control of a three-messenger system, also called the hypothalamic-pituitary-thyroid axis. The hypothalamus produces two hormones: TRH and somatostatin. TRH has a stimulatory effect, whereas somatostatin has an inhibitory effect on the pituitary. TSH produced in the anterior pituitary is the major controller of the production and release of thyroid hormones. Negative feedback is exerted by thyroid hormones on the pituitary and hypothalamus [17]. Thyroid hormone stimulates almost all aspects of carbohydrate metabolism, including rapid uptake of glucose by the cells, enhanced glycolysis, enhanced gluconeogenesis, increased rate of absorption from the gastrointestinal tract, and increased insulin secretion with its resultant effects on carbohydrate metabolism. Thyroid hormones are also the key controllers of the part of metabolic heat production that is necessary for the maintenance of high and constant body temperature [20].

Thyroid hormones influence growth and differentiation/maturation of birds. Growth involves mainly cell proliferation but also may result from increases in cell size. Thyroid hormones are important in triggering tissue-specific differentiation and maturation processes in many tissues. Some studies suggest that thyroid hormones are necessary for the development of normal brain architecture and neuronal connections critical to the function of brain regions [21]. Thyroid hormones are important in hatching, molting, and reproduction in birds. Thyroid hormones are necessary for reproductive system development and reproduction function, but extremely high levels have been shown to have antigonadal effects. Thyroid hormones and starvation can be used to induce molt, and alterations in plasma thyroid hormones occur in conjunction with natural molts [17].

There are environmental influences on thyroid function. The factors that have the greatest influence seem to be changes in temperature and food availability. Environmental cold can act through the HPT axis to increase thyroid release and can alter the conversion of T_4 to T_3. Alterations in food availability and composition also alter thyroid status; food restriction decreases circulating T_3, whereas feeding increases it [17].

The parathyroid gland

Anatomy

The parathyroid gland is a small gland located immediately behind the thyroid gland. The number of parathyroid glands in birds varies between two and four. They are encapsulated by connective tissue and composed mainly of chief cells. The content is consistent with a low level of parathyroid hormone (PTH) secretion [22]. Removal of the parathyroid gland causes hypocalcemia, tetany, and, ultimately, death and hypophosphatemia in some species [23].

Physiology

Birds are sensitive to PTH. The primary targets of PTH in birds are bone and the kidneys, as in mammals. The major stimulus for PTH secretion from the chief cells is a fall in plasma Ca^{2+} concentration, whereas a rise in Ca^{2+} suppresses it [24]. PTH has two effects on bone in causing absorption of calcium and phosphate. One is rapid phase, which begins in minutes and increases progressively over several hours. This effect results from activation of the already existing bones cells, mainly osteocytes, to promote calcium and phosphate absorption. The second phase is much slower and requires several days, even weeks. This phase results from the proliferation of the osteoclasts, followed by increased osteoclastic reabsorption of the bone itself [23].

The effect PTH has on the kidneys is that it increases glomerular filtration rate, urine flow rate, and P_i and Ca^{2+} clearance. Studies show that renal Ca^{2+} and P_i homeostasis in chickens depends on a balanced release of PTH and calcitonin. The response time in chickens is much faster than it is in mammals, but this response is less effective when Ca^{2+} demands are high, as in growing or egg-laying birds [23].

The ultimobranchial glands

Anatomy

Birds possess anatomically distinct, asymmetrically paired ultimobranchial glands, which in chickens lie posterior to the parathyroid glands and caudodorsal to the base of the brachiocephalic artery into the common carotid and subclavian arteries [22].

Physiology

The avian ultimobranchial gland is rich in calcitonin, the principal cell having a marked resemblance to mammalian C cells. Calcitonin secretion is regulated primarily by rising plasma Ca^{2+} levels, which lead to increased secretion from the C cells. Calcitonin levels are higher in adult male chickens than in egg-laying female chickens except for a brief period immediately before the commencement of laying. The role of calcitonin in bone and Ca metabolism still remains a mystery. Only in mammalian species has it been shown to regulate plasma Ca levels, the basis of its hypocalcemic action lying in an ability to inhibit osteoclastic reabsorption [25].

The uropygial gland and the vitamin D system

Anatomy

The uropygial gland, or preen gland, is a bilobed holocrine gland located dorsally at the base of the trunk. It is the principal cutaneous gland of birds. It is present in most species, excluding the ostrich, emu, cassowary, many pigeons, and certain species of psittacines. Among the psittacine species that do not possess a preen gland are the hyacinth macaw (*Anodorhynchus hyacinthinus*) the Lear's macaw (*Anodorhynchus leari*), and the Spix's macaw (*Cyanopsitta spixii*). All of the parrots in the genus *Amazona* also do not possess a preen gland. The gland is present in canaries and most finches.

It is usually drained by a pair of ducts, each of which drains one lobe and opens into a single, narrow papilla [26].

Physiology

A study done in 1931 reported that the removal of the uropygial gland causes rickets in chicks, even when they are fed a healthy diet and exposed to sunlight. The researcher concluded that birds must secrete provitamin D_3 from the preen gland onto their feathers, where it is converted into vitamin D_3. It has since been well established that chickens metabolize vitamin D_3 to 25-(OH)-D_3 and 1,25-(OH)$_2D_3$ in their liver and kidneys, respectively [27]. Birds, however, discriminate between vitamin D_2 and D_3, unlike their mammalian counterparts. Chickens are able to use vitamin D_2 and D_3 because avian plasma vitamin D–binding protein has a low affinity for vitamin D_2, thus it is broken down more rapidly [27].

The kidney synthesizes and secretes 1,25-(OH)$_2D_3$, and numerous factors stimulate its production, including PTH, 1,25-(OH)$_2D_3$ itself, and prolactin. Vitamin D and its metabolites are transported in association with plasma albumins and, in some avian species, with α- and β-globulins. 1,25(OH)$_2D_3$ plays an important role in Ca^{2+} and bone metabolism. In the intestines, 1,25(OH)$_2D_3$ regulates absorption of Ca^{2+} by inducing RNA transcription and synthesis of proteins, the most important being calbindin D_{28k}. The physiologic function of calbindin D_{28k} has not been well established, but in vitamin D-deficient birds, intestinal calbindin mRNA is barely detectable and increases dramatically after an injection of 1,25-(OH)$_2D_3$. A similar—if not identical—protein has been found in the avian uterus [28].

1,25-(OH)$_2D_3$ seems to facilitate bone formation by inducing biosynthesis of osteocalcin, a binding protein. The function of this noncollagenous vitamin D–binding protein in skeletal mineralization is still somewhat of a mystery, but it seems to be a specific product of osteoblasts during bone formation [23].

The adrenal glands

Anatomy

The adrenal glands are paired organs located anteriorly and medially to the cephalic lobe of the kidney. Their shape is generally flattened and they lie close together, even fusing in some species. The glands receive arterial blood from the cranial renal arteries and occasionally from the aorta, and each gland drains into the caudal vena cava [29]. Preganglionic and postganglionic sympathetic fibers innervate the chromaffin cells. Preganglionic sympathetic fibers from the thoracic and synsacral splanchnic nerves converge on the cranial and caudal ganglia located on the pericapsular sheath. Some researchers suggest that the avian adrenal gland is also innervated by parasympathetic fibers, presumably from the vagus nerve via the celiac plexus [30].

The pineal gland

Anatomy

The avian epiphysis cerebri, or pineal gland, is located at the dorsal surface of the brain between the telencephalon and the cerebellum. It consists of a distal enlargement, the pineal vesicle, which adheres to the dura mater, and a proximal stalk. Most diurnally active birds have a well-developed pineal gland. Rudimentary pineal glands have been found in some nocturnal and crepuscular species [31]. The pineal gland is connected to the brain via afferent and efferent pathways. The gland is richly innervated by sympathetic postganglionic fibers that originate in the superior cervical ganglia [31].

Physiology

Melatonin is the most significant hormone produced by the pineal gland; it is also produced in the retina, the Harderian gland, and the gastrointestinal tract [31]. This extrapineal melatonin is not released into the vascular system; instead it acts near the site of production. Pineal melatonin is released into systemic circulation. A characteristic feature of pineal melatonin production and secretion is a 24-hour rhythm, with levels being higher at night. The functions of melatonin in many vertebrates include involvement in thermoregulation, skin color changes, reproduction, immune response, puberty, sleep regulation, aging, and circadian organization. Of all these functions, only a few have been established in birds, including circadian organization, thermoregulation, and sleep regulation [31].

There are three parts to the avian circadian system: the pineal gland, the avian equivalent to the mammalian suprachiasmatic nucleus, and the eyes. Studies have found that these three features are connected with each other in a neuroendocrine feedback loop and that the gross output of this composite pacemaking system depends on inhibitory interactions among the three components. In other words, the components synchronize and amplify each other through resonance [31].

Periodically changing environmental factors, such as food availability, temperature, and social stimuli, can synchronize avian circadian rhythms, but the most important synchronizer of circadian rhythms is the periodic alterations of light intensity [32]. In birds, light for circadian synchronization is perceived in part by the eyes, from which photic information is transmitted to the suprachiasmatic nucleus via the retinohypothalamic tract. Light perceived by the pineal and deep encephalic photoreceptors also may play a role in synchronization [33]. The life of most birds is organized not only on a daily basis but also on a yearly basis. Annual cycles in reproduction and other processes are strongly controlled by the seasonal changes in day length. There is little evidence, however, of a significant contribution of the pineal gland in generating circannual cycles [34].

Melatonin has been shown to reduce body temperature and metabolic rate in some species of birds. It also has been shown to be involved with sleep regulation, which is believed to be done by synchronizing the physiology of birds to the external light-dark cycle, which reduces energy expenditure during periods of inactivity [35].

The pancreas

Anatomy

The avian pancreas lies suspended between the ascending and descending duodenum, conveniently located to contribute its hormonal mix to the portal vein. In most birds it is composed of three lobes: dorsal, ventral, and splenic, with the dorsal and ventral lobes remaining separate in pigeons and ducks. The endocrine portion of the avian pancreas occupies considerably more tissue mass than in mammals, and the distribution of cell types differs. Three types of islets are described that vary according to lobar location and species. The dark islets are comprised mostly of A cells and the light islets contain a mixture of B and D cells. The third type, the mixed islets, has all three cell types: A, B, and D cells. The dark islets are irregularly shaped, large, and indistinctly separated from the exocrine pancreatic tissue. By contrast, the light islets are round to elliptical in shape, compact, and distinct from the exocrine tissue [21]. A cells synthesize and release glucagon; B cells synthesize and release insulin; D cells secrete somatostatin.

Summary

A detailed understanding of the anatomy and physiology of the avian endocrine system enables clinicians to make better clinical judgments and improve diagnostic methods, resulting in better treatment of endocrine diseases. Knowledge of the uniqueness of an individual species on a biochemical level is vital to successful therapy.

References

[1] Scanes CG. Introduction to endocrinology: pituitary gland. In: Whittow GC, editor. Sturkie's avian physiology. 5th edition. San Diego (CA): Academic; 2000. p. 437–60.
[2] Lumeij JT. Endocrinology. In: Altman RB, Clubb SL, Dorrestein GM, et al, editors. Avian medicine and surgery. Philadelphia: W.B. Saunders; 1997. p. 582–605.
[3] Sharp PJ, Klandorf H. Environmental and physiological factors controlling thyroid function in galliforms. In: Follett BK, Ishii S, Chandoloa A, editors. The endocrine system and the environment. Berlin: Springer-Verlag; 1985. p. 175–81.

[4] Almeida OF, Thomas DH. Effects of feeding pattern on the pituitary thyroid axis in the Japanese quail. Gen Comp Endocrinol 1981;44:508–13.

[5] Berghman LR, Lens P, Decuypere E, et al. Glycosylated chicken growth hormone. Gen Comp Endocrinol 1987;68:408–14.

[6] Guyton AC, Hall JE. Pituitary hormones and their control by the hypothalamus. In: Textbook of medical physiology. 11th edition. Philadelphia: Elsevier Saunders; 2006. p. 918–43.

[7] Houston B, O'Neill IE. Insulin and growth hormone act synergistically to stimulate insulin-like growth factor-I production by cultured chicken hepatocytes. J Endocrinol 1990;128:389–93.

[8] McCann-Levorse LM, Radecki SV, Donoghue DJ, et al. Ontogeny of pituitary growth hormone and growth hormone mRNA in the chicken. Proceedings of the Society for Experimental Biology and Medicine 1993;202:109–113.

[9] Buntin JD, Ruzychi E, Witebsky J. Prolactin receptors in dove brain: autoradiographic analysis of binding characteristics in discrete brain regions and accessibility to blood-borne prolactin. Neuroendocrinology 1993;57:738–50.

[10] Carisa RV, Scanes CG, Malamed S. Isolated adrenocortical cells of the domestic fowl (Gallus domesticus): steroidogenic and ultrastructural properties. J Steroid Biochem 1985; 22:273–9.

[11] Jozsa R, Vigh S, Schally AV, et al. Localization of corticotropin-releasing factor-containing neurons in the brain of the domestic fowl. Cell Tissue Res 1984;236:245–8.

[12] Acher R, Chauvet J, Chauvet MT. Phylogeny of the neurohypophyseal hormones: the avian active peptides. Eur J Biochem 1970;17:509–13.

[13] Shirley HV, Nalbandov AV. Effects of neurohypophysectomy in domestic chickens. Endocrinology 1956;58:477–83.

[14] Saito N, Kinzler S, Koike TI. Arginine vasotocin and mesotocin levels in theca and granulosa levels of the ovary during the oviposition cycle in hens (Gallus domesticus). Gen Comp Endocrinol 1990;79:54–63.

[15] Koike TI, Shimada K, Cornett LE. Plasma levels of immunoreactive mesotocin and vasotocin during oviposition in chickens: relationship to oxytocic action of the peptides in vitro and peptide interaction with myometrial membrane binding sites. Gen Comp Endocrinol 1988; 70:119–26.

[16] Robinzon B, Koike TI, Neldon HL, et al. Distribution of immunoreactive mesotocin and vasotocin in the brain and pituitary of chickens. Peptides 1988;9:829–33.

[17] McNabb FMA. Thyroids. In: Whittow GC, editor. Sturkie's avian physiology. 5th edition. San Diego (CA): Academic; 2000. p. 461–71.

[18] Astier H. Thyroid gland in birds: structure and function. In: Epple A, Stetson MH, editors. Avian endocrinology. New York: Academic Press; 1980. p. 167–89.

[19] Chanoine JP, Alex S, Fang SL, et al. Role of transthyretin in the transport of thyroxine from the blood of the choroids plexus, the cerebrospinal fluid, and the brain. Endocrinology 1992; 130:933–8.

[20] Danforth E Jr, Burger A. The role of thyroid hormones in the control of energy expenditure. Clin Endocrinol Metab 1984;13:581–95.

[21] Oglesbee BL, Orosz S, Dorrestein GM, et al. The endocrine system. In: Altman RB, Clubb SL, Dorrestein GM, editors. Avian medicine and surgery. Philadelphia: WB Saunders; 1997. p. 475–88.

[22] Kenny AD. Parathyroid and ultimobranchial glands. In: Sturkie PD, editor. Avian physiology. 4th edition. New York: Springer-Verlag; 1986.

[23] Dacke CG. The parathyroids, calcitonin, and vitamin D. In: Whittow GC, editor. Sturkie's avian physiology. 5th edition. San Diego (CA): Academic; 2000. p. 473–88.

[24] Brown EM. Extracellular Ca^{2+} sensing, regulation of parathyroid cell function and role of Ca^{2+} and other ions as extracellular (first) messengers. Physiol Rev 1991;71:371–411.

[25] Copp DH, Kline LW. Calcitonin. In: Pang PKT, Schreibman MP, editors. Vertebrate endocrinology fundamentals and biomedical implications, vol. 3. New York: Academic Press; 1989. p. 79–103.

[26] King AS, McLelland J. Birds: their structure and function. London: Bailliere Tindall; 1984. p. 286–90.

[27] Holick MF. Phylogenetic and evolutionary aspects of vitamin D from phytoplankton to humans. In: Pang PKT, Schreibman MG, editors. Vertebrate endocrinology, vol. 3. New York: Academic Press; 1989. p. 7–43.

[28] Fullmer CS, Bridak ME, Bar A, et al. The purification of calcium binding protein from the uterus of laying hens. Proceedings of the Society for Experimental Biology and Medicine 1976;152:237–41.

[29] Chester Jones I. The adrenal cortex. London/New York: Cambridge University Press; 1957.

[30] Carsia RV, Harvey S. Adrenals. In: Whittow GC, editor. Sturkie's avian physiology. 5th edition. San Diego (CA): Academic; 2000. p. 489–537.

[31] Gwinner E, Hau M. The pineal gland, circadian rhythms, and photoperiodism. In: Whittow GC, editor. Sturkie's avian physiology. 5th edition. San Diego: Academic; 2000. p. 557–68.

[32] Ashoff J. Free-running and entrained circadian rhythms. In: Aschoff J, editor. Handbook of behavioural neurobiology, vol. 4. New York/London: Plenum; 1981. p. 81–93.

[33] Cassone VM, Menaker M. Is the avian circadian system a neuroendocrine loop? J Exp Zool 1984;232:539–49.

[34] Gwinner E. Melatonin and the circadian system of birds: model of internal resonance. In: Hiroshige T, Honma K, editors. Circadian clocks and ecology. Sapporo: Hokkaido University Press; 1989.

[35] Berger RJ, Phillips NH. Constant light suppresses sleep and circadian rhythms in pigeons without consequent sleep rebound in darkness. Am J Physiol 1994;36:R945–52.

VETERINARY
CLINICS
Exotic Animal Practice

Vet Clin Exot Anim 11 (2008) 15–23

The Avian Thyroid Gland

Robert E. Schmidt, DVM, PhD, DACVP[a],*,
Drury R. Reavill, DVM, DABVP–Avian, DACVP[b]

[a]Zoo/Exotic Pathology Service, PO Box 267, Greenview, CA 96037, USA
[b]7647 Wachtel Way, Citrus Heights, CA 96037, USA

There has been a considerable amount of research regarding the function of the avian thyroid gland, particularly in chickens. There is also more information on diseases of the avian thyroid gland, although it is usually in the form of case reports. This article covers a limited amount of material on the structure and function of the avian thyroid gland and its diseases.

Embryology and anatomy

The full endocrine system is developed during the embryonic stages of the domestic fowl and probably in all avian species [1]. The thyroid glands arise from the floor of the pharynx in the area of the first and second pharyngeal pouches [2]. The hypothalamus, pituitary, and thyroid glands of the developing chick embryo synthesize their appropriate hormones early in development (ie, before day 5.5 of incubation) [3]. In adult birds the thyroids are paired and lie just cranial to the thoracic inlet. They are lateral to the trachea and medial to the jugular veins [4]. Histologically, thyroid glands contain numerous follicles lined by low cuboidal epithelium (Fig. 1). Colloid is present in the follicles as an amorphous eosinophilic material. Birds do not have C cells (parafollicular cells that store substantial amounts of calcitonin in their cytoplasm) in their thyroid glands. Calcitonin is produced by the ultimobranchial bodies that are located as separate glandular structures caudal to the thyroid glands and adjacent to the parathyroid glands [5].

Thyroid physiology

Synthesis of thyroid hormones occurs in birds when iodide is concentrated within the thyroid gland by the maintenance of a gradient over

---

* Corresponding author.
E-mail address: zooexotic@sisqtel.net (R.E. Schmidt).

doi:10.1016/j.cvex.2007.09.008
vetexotic.theclinics.com

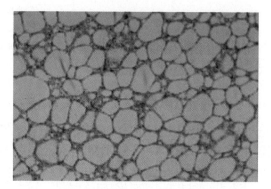

Fig. 1. A photomicrograph of a normal avian thyroid.

that of blood [6]. Iodide is converted to I_2 and then I^+. Iodine concentration in the avian thyroid peaks at 6 hours and is then stored for several days [7].

Avian thyroglobulin is highly iodinated, and the iodine represents 1.5% thyroglobulin by weight [8]. A peroxidase system converts iodide to iodine, with a second enzyme system combining iodinated tyrosines with thyroglobulin to form tri-iodothyronine (T_3) and thyroxine (T_4) [6]. Intrathyroidal iodination and deiodination occur continually, leading to randomization of thyroidal iodine, which shifts between tyrosine and thyronine randomly [9].

Control of thyroid hormone production is via a negative feedback loop regulated by the hypothalamus and adenohypophysis [6]. A decrease in circulating T_3 (for any reason) below metabolic requirements stimulates the anterior pituitary to release thyroid-stimulating hormone (TSH). In adult chickens, thyroid-releasing hormone (TRH) does not cause TSH release [10]. Exogenous administration of T_4 can lead to a decrease in TSH. Secretion of TSH is controlled by the hypothalamus via the indirect action of TRH. The hypothalamus secretes TRH during stress, hypothermia, febrile illness, and periods of decreased circulating thyroid hormones. TRH secreted by the hypothalamus is not thyrotrophic; rather it increases the release of growth hormone by the pituitary gland. Growth hormone then increases T_3 by stimulating the monodeiodination of T_4. In birds, thyroid hormones and growth hormones are related because thyroid hormones inhibit synthesis and release of growth hormone [11,12]. Growth hormone seems to impair T_4 release and stimulates its monodeiodination [10,11].

In birds, TSH is mainly thyrotrophic, with no influence on peripheral activation of T_4-T_3 [13]. TSH stimulates the proliferation, differentiation, and metabolism of thyroid follicle cells. Under the influence of TSH, cyclic $3',5'$ adenosine monophosphate (cAMP) is activated in thyroid follicular epithelial cells. Increased cAMP leads to increased iodide trapping from the blood by the follicular cells [14]. As a result, follicular colloid is processed into follicular epithelial cells, which leads to release of thyroid hormones into the circulation. Approximately 60% is T_4, and 40% is T_3 (the biologically active form). In the liver, T_4 and T_3 are metabolized through the action of I 5' deiodinase [6,15]. Growth hormone inhibits type III deiodinating enzyme in the liver, which results in the previously described increases of T_3. Other hormones, such as follicle-stimulating hormone, can increase follicular diameter and epithelial cell height of the thyroid gland in immature chickens [16].

Thyroid hormones control metabolism and development with the actions mediated by nuclear thyroid hormone receptors, which have the highest affinity for T_3. T_3 circulates in the blood bound to prealbumin and albumin and is metabolized by the liver and kidney. Compared with mammals, it has a shorter half-life.

External influences on thyroid function

Young and adult chickens secrete T_4 in the summer at half of the winter rate [6]. This effect is directly correlated to ambient temperature. In winter, the follicular cells are more columnar and follicular volume is greater [17]. Photoperiod also affects thyroid function and metabolism. A long photoperiod depresses I^{131} uptake in ducks and quail [6]. Long days inhibit thyroid function but stimulate thyrotrophic activity. During daylight, T_4 is depressed and T_3 is elevated, whereas the reverse occurs at night [18].

Thyroid hormone is involved in maintaining photorefractoriness in turkey hens [19]. In male turkeys, light intensity affects food conversion efficiency, with body weight highest under the lowest light intensity, which coincides with higher weight gain and lower food intake [20]. Food intake and diet composition are also related to thyroid hormone concentration and metabolism. The T_4/T_3 ratio increases during fasting, and plasma TSH concentration decreases [21,22]. Hypothalamic TRH content is elevated, which suggests a decreased hypothalamic release. Fasting also can lead to increased hepatic type III deiodinase (D3) and decreased renal D3 activity. No change was noted in either hepatic or renal type I deiodinase (D1) [23].

The level of dietary protein fed to chickens had an effect on the concentrations of T_4 and T_3 after adding T_3 to the birds' diet. With a high level of protein, T_4 was greater and T_3 was less; however, the protein level did not change the response to the addition of T_3 to the diet, which indicated that dietary protein levels may not affect adaptive responses to T_3 [24]. The effect may be caused by selected amino acid deficits [25]. When chicks are fed a restricted diet there is a decrease in plasma T_3. Arginine deficiency prevents this decrease but does not alter T_4 concentration, which suggests that there is a specific alteration in the metabolism of T_3. Methionine deficiency also leads to elevated plasma T_3 concentration in diet-restricted chicks.

Other amino acids with similar effects include lysine and isoleucine. Leucine and threonine have no effect on plasma T_3. Lysine is the only amino acid that lowers T_4. The level of selenium affects the growth of chickens via thyroid hormone metabolism [26]. Dietary selenium supplementation increases plasma T_3, whereas T_4 decreases. Hepatic 5' deiodinase activity is elevated by selenium, and a selenium deficiency can depress growth by inhibiting 5' deiodinase activity, which causes lower plasma T_3 concentration.

Thyroid function after hatching

Immunocytochemical studies and more traditional techniques, such as gland ablation and hormone replacement, have revealed the time of appearance of each hormone in the axis, the relative amounts of hormone present in each gland at different developmental stages, and a general picture of the pattern of maturation of the hypothalamic-pituitary-thyroid axis. Studies of the pituitary control of thyroglobulin remain limited by the lack of adequately specific techniques for measuring avian TSH. Our understanding of peripheral thyroid hormone dynamics is progressing as a result of iodothyronine deiodinase assays, but full understanding requires more elaborate studies that adequately characterize the enzyme systems [27]. Precocial and altricial modes of avian development have different degrees of maturation and physiologic capabilities at hatching. In precocial birds, thyroid function and its control are well developed during the latter part of incubation. Hatchlings have metabolic responses to cooling and relatively mature sensory and locomotor capabilities. In altricial birds, thyroid function has minimal maturation until after hatch [28].

Intracellular thyroid hormone availability is influenced by different metabolic pathways. Some of the changes in intracellular thyroid hormone availability can be linked to changes in local deiodination and sulfation capacities. The chicken thyroid secretes predominantly T_4, whereas thyroid hormone receptors preferentially bind 3,5,3' T_3. The metabolism of T_4 secreted by the thyroid gland in peripheral tissues, which leads to the production and degradation of receptor-active T_3, plays a major role in thyroid function [29]. Because the avian thyroid gland secretes almost exclusively T_4, the availability of receptor-active 3,3',5 T_3 is regulated in the extrathyroidal tissues, essentially by deiodination. Like most other vertebrates, birds possess three types of iodothyronine deiodinases (D1, D2, and D3) that closely resemble their mammalian counterparts. Deiodination in birds is regulated by hormones from several endocrine axes, including thyroid hormones, growth hormone, and glucocorticoids. Deiodination is also influenced by external parameters, such as nutrition, temperature, light, and environmental pollutants [30].

Thyroid function tests

Thyroid scintigraphy was conducted in normal and radiothyroidectomized cockatiels using sodium technetium Tc 99m pertechnetate. Scintigraphy was capable of detecting thyroid hypofunction [31]. This test is a research tool, however, and not readily available to practitioners. The best method of testing the avian thyroid for abnormalities involves the administration of TSH and measuring the serum T_4 concentration after a particular time period [32,33]. Unfortunately, veterinary TSH is no longer on the market, and the test must be done with an expensive human product [34].

The alternative is measurement of T_4 only [35]. Because avian T_4 is lower than mammalian, the test must be able to detect lower T_4 values. A single, low T_4 test result cannot lead to a definitive diagnosis of hypothyroidism, and a single, normal result may not be proof that the bird does not have hypothyroidism. The test should be interpreted in association with multiple factors, including clinical signs and other tests.

Recently, a method for using a high-sensitivity radioimmunoassay to measure total T_4 concentration was developed [36]. This method was developed using psittacine birds only. In these birds it is a way to measure T_4 concentrations. Results of the study indicated that T_4 concentrations in blue-fronted Amazon parrots were higher and more variable than in other species tested.

Diseases of the thyroid gland

Diseases of the thyroid are most completely documented in chickens but are less well described in other avian species. Various conditions have been reported, but overt clinical disease is uncommon. Cystic thyroids are occasionally seen, but the cysts actually may arise in the ultimobranchial body [37]. A partial persistence of the thyroglossal duct can lead to cysts lined by epithelium similar to that of thyroid follicles [38].

The immune system may be affected by the thyroid gland. The gland may play a part in humoral immunity, with physiologic levels of thyroid hormone being necessary to maintain normal weights of the spleen and bursa of Fabricius [39]. The thyroid also is involved in autoimmune diseases in obese strain chickens, which get a spontaneous autoimmune thyroiditis [40,41]. The condition develops in the first 2 to 3 weeks after hatching. As in humans, the iodine content of obese chickens' thyroglobulin was lower than that of normal chickens; however, these chickens have almost no inorganic iodide in their thyroid glands. A recent review of spontaneous chicken models for human autoimmune diseases described the obese strain, which has a Hashimoto-like autoimmune thyroiditis [42]. A morphologically similar condition has been seen in African gray parrots [38,43]. Grossly affected glands are usually small, pale, and irregular. Variable follicular collapse associated with lymphoid cell infiltration, lymphoid follicle formation, and mild connective tissue proliferation may be seen histologically.

The most common avian thyroid problem reported is hyperplasia (goiter) [44]. Although the literature indicates that the condition is most common in budgerigars, a study of 16 years of our data indicated that macaws, particularly blue and gold macaws, have the highest incidence of hyperplastic goiter [45]. Colloid goiter is also seen sporadically [46]. It may be the involutionary stage of hyperplasia with grossly enlarged glands that histologically have large colloid-filled follicles lined by cuboidal or flattened epithelial cells. Clinical signs of thyroid hyperplasia may be absent or are referable to bilateral enlargement of the thyroid glands, which put pressure on surrounding tissues, including the trachea. Grossly there is bilateral thyroid enlargement, with the glands being red-brown or purple [46,47], and histologically numerous follicles are lined by enlarged epithelial cells (Fig. 2). Colloid is minimal or absent. The primary cause of goiter in budgerigars has been considered to be iodine deficiency [44], but other potential causes include the feeding of goitrogenic substances of plant origin and genetically induced biosynthetic problems [45].

Functional hypothyroidism is considered uncommon in birds [48], although one case in a scarlet macaw was documented [49]. We have seen a documented case with severe feather loss, epidermal atrophy, and no inflammatory skin changes. Disturbances in thyroid hormone production may affect molting and feather growth. In penguins, changes in T_3 were not shown to be consistent with molting, but increased T_4 and a decrease in plasma levels of sex steroid hormones induced molting [50]. In thyroidectomized birds (spotted munia) T_4 seems to be more effective than T_3 at inducing feather regeneration [51]. In chickens, doses of T_4 at 0.2 mg/bird diminished egg production but did not result in molting, whereas doses of 0.4 mg/bird caused feather loss after day 14 of administration [52]. In general, an increase in thyroid hormones leads to molting, possibly by stimulating new feather growth [53]. Because of the difficulties in thyroid testing, correlating T_4 levels with feather problems seen in pet birds is not usually done, and the role that the thyroid plays in clinical disease in pet birds is not well documented.

An experimental model of hypothyroidism was developed in cockatiels [54]; however, classic clinical and laboratory signs, such as poor feathering and hypercholesterolemia, were either absent or mild 48 days after radiothyroidectomy. This finding may indicate that a longer course of the disease

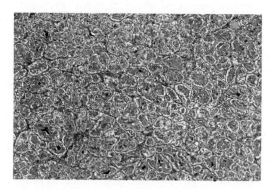

Fig. 2. A photomicrograph of a thyroid hyperplasia with marked proliferation of follicular epithelial cells and loss of colloid.

is necessary for these signs to develop. Without TSH response testing or histologic confirmation of lesions associated with clinical hypothyroidism, the true incidence of hypothyroidism is difficult to determine. In older, obese Amazon parrots, lesions of the thyroid have been associated with atherosclerosis; hypothyroidism was suspected but not confirmed [44]. In our series [45], hypothyroidism was considered a possible stress factor leading to other diseases, but it was not proved by appropriate clinical testing.

Thyroid neoplasia, including adenoma and carcinoma, are frequently reported in budgerigars and may cause respiratory signs caused by pressure on the trachea [55]. Tumors are also seen in other species [46]. From our case files, tumors of the thyroid gland, including adenomas and carcinomas, are more frequently identified with cockatiels. Other species having thyroid adenoma include Maribu storks, Japanese quail, lilac crown Amazon parrots, orange wing Amazon parrots, and budgies. Carcinomas were identified in a Hyacinth macaw, lilac crown Amazon, black-headed Caique, African gray parrot, and several budgies. When clinical signs were noted, there was the presence of a mass in the neck or crop dysfunction. Thyroid adenocarcinoma was diagnosed in an adult bald eagle (*Haliaeetus leukocephalus*) that had clinical signs of weakness and inability to fly. Radiographs revealed a large, soft tissue mass in the area of the left coracoid and clavicular bones. At necropsy, a large mass was noted within the interclavicular air sac. It had histologic features that were consistent with thyroid adenocarcinoma [56]. Grossly, carcinomas may vary in size and can be irregular and pale. Histologically, adenomas are comprised of large cuboidal epithelial cells that form follicular and papillary structures and cystic spaces. Carcinomas are similar but more anaplastic and invasive [57]. The tumors usually are not functionally secreting [44].

The thyroid gland is not uncommonly involved with systemic diseases. The most common disease, primarily in non-psittacines, involves amyloid deposition. From our case files, anseriformes and ciconiformes (flamingos) had amyloid identified in multiple organs, including the thyroid gland.

References

[1] Scanes CG, Hart LE, Decuypere E, et al. Endocrinology of the avian embryo: an overview. J Exp Zool Suppl 1987;1:253–64.
[2] King AS, McLelland J. Endocrine system. In: Birds: their structure and function. London: Bailliere Tindall; 1984. p. 204–13.
[3] Thommes RC. Ontoenesis of thyroid function and regulation in the developing chick embryo. J Exp Zool Suppl 1987;1:273–9.
[4] O'Malley B. Avian anatomy and physiology. In: Clinical anatomy and physiology of exotic species. Edinburg (IL): Elsevier; 2005. p. 144–5.
[5] Banks WJ. Endocrine system. In: Applied veterinary histology. St. Louis (MO): Mosby; 1993. p. 414–28.
[6] Wentworth BC, Ringer RK. Thyroids. In: Sturkie PD, editor. Avian physiology. New York: Springer-Verlag; 1985. p. 452–65.

[7] Newcomer WS. Dietary iodine and accumulation of radioiodine in thyroids of chickens. Am J Physiol 1978;234:168–76.

[8] Hoshiro T, Ui N. Comparative studies on the properties of thyroglobulins from various animal species. Endocrinol Jpn 1970;17:521–33.

[9] Newcomer WS. Accumulation of radioiodine in thiouracil-hyperplastic thyroids of chicks. Am J Physiol 1979;237:147–51.

[10] Kuhn ER, Berghman LR, Moons L, et al. Hypothalamic and peripheral control of thyroid function during the life cycle of the chicken. In: Sharp PJ, editor. Avian endocrinology. London: Burgess Science; 1993. p. 29–46.

[11] Hull KL, Janssens WCJ, Baumbach WR, et al. Thyroid glands: novel sites of growth hormone action. J Endocrinol 1995;146:449–58.

[12] McNabb FM. Thyroid hormones, their activation, degradation and effects on metabolism. J Nutr 1995;125(6 Suppl):1773S–6S.

[13] Singh PP, Pradeep Kumar G, Laloraya M. Regulation of superoxide anion radical-superoxide dismutase system in the avian thyroid by TSH with reference to thyroid hormogenesis. Biochem Biophys Res Commun 1997;239:212–6.

[14] Larsen PR, Davies TF, Hay ID. The thyroid gland. In: Wilson JD, Foster DW, editors. Williams textbook of endocrinology. 9th editon. Philadelphia: WB Saunders; 1998. p. 390–414.

[15] Kohrle J, Brabant G, Hesch RD. Metabolism of thyroid hormones. Horm Res 1987;26: 58–78.

[16] Dobozy O, Balkanyi L, Csaba G. Overlapping effect of thyroid stimulating hormone and follicle stimulating hormone on the thyroid gland in baby chickens. Acta Physiol Acad Sci Hung 1981;57:171–5.

[17] Breit S, Konig HE, Stoger E. The morphology of the thyroid gland in poultry with special regard to seasonal variations. Anat Histol Embryol 1998;27:271–6.

[18] Klundorf H, Lea W, Sharp PJ. Thyroid function in laying, incubating and broody bantam hens. Gen Comp Endocrinol 1982;47:492–6.

[19] Siopes T. Transient hypothyroidism reinitiates egg laying in turkey breeder hens: termination of photorefractoriness by propylthiouracil. Poult Sci 1997;76:1776–82.

[20] Yahav S, Hruwitz S, Rozenboim I. The effect of light intensity on growth and development of turkey toms. Br Poult Sci 2000;41:101–6.

[21] May JD, Reece FN. Relationship of photoperiod and feed intake to thyroid hormone concentration. Poult Sci 1986;65:801–6.

[22] Geris KL, Berghman LR, Kuhn ER, et al. The drop in plasma thyrotropin concentrations in fasted chickens is caused by an actin at the level of the hypothalamus: role of corticosterone. Domest Anim Endocrinol 1999;16:231–7.

[23] Van der Geyten S, Van Rompaey E, Sanders JP, et al. Regulation of thyroid hormone metabolism during fasting and refeeding in chickens. Gen Comp Endocrinol 1999;116:272–80.

[24] Rosebrough RW, McMurtry JP, Vasilatos-Younken R. Dietary protein effects on the broiler's adaptation to triiodothyronine. Growth Dev Aging 1999;63:85–98.

[25] Carew LB, Evarts KG, Alster FA. Growth and plasma thyroid hormone concentrations of chicks fed diets deficient in essential amino acids. Poult Sci 1997;76:1398–404.

[26] Jianhua H, Ohtsuka A, Hayashi K. Selenium influences growth via thyroid hormone status in broiler chickens. Br J Nutr 2000;84:727–32.

[27] McNabb FM. Thyroid function in embryonic and early posthatch chickens and quail. Poult Sci 1989;68:990–8.

[28] McNabb FM. Avian thyroid development and adaptive plasticity. Gen Comp Endocrinol 2006;147:93–101.

[29] Decuypere E, Van ASP, Van der Geyten S, et al. Thyroid hormone availability and activity in avian species: a review. Domest Anim Endocrinol 2005;29:63–77.

[30] Darras VM, Verhoelst CHJ, Reyns GE, et al. Thyroid hormone deiodination in birds. Thyroid 2006;16:25–35.

[31] Harms CA, Hoskinson JJ, Bruyette DS, et al. Technetium-99m and iodine-131 thyroid scintigraphy in normal and radiothyroidectomized cockatiels [*Nymphicus hollandicus*]. Vet Radiol Ultrasound 1994;35:473–8.

[32] Zenoble RD, Kemppainen RJ, Young DW, et al. Endocrine response of healthy parrots to ACTH and thyroid stimulating hormone. J Am Vet Assoc 1985;187:1116–8.

[33] Lothrop CD, Loomis MR, Olsen JH. Thyrotropin stimulation test for evaluation of thyroid function in psittacine birds. J Am Vet Assoc 1985;186:47–8.

[34] Fudge AM, Speer B. Selected controversial topics in avian diagnostic testing. Sem Av Exotic Pet Med 2001;10:96–101.

[35] Rae M. Avian endocrine disorders. In: Fudge AM, editor. Laboratory medicine: avian and exotic pets. Philadelphia: Saunders; 2000. p. 76–89.

[36] Greenacre CB, Young DW, Behrend EN, et al. Validation of a novel high-sensitivity radio-immunoassay procedure for measurement of total thyroxine concentration in psittacine birds and snakes. Am J Vet Res 2001;62:1750–4.

[37] Ito M, Kameda Y, Tagawa T. An ultrastructural study of the cysts in chicken ultimobranchial glands, with special reference to C-cells. Cell Tissue Res 1986;246:39–44.

[38] Schmidt RE, Reavill DR, Phalen DN. Endocrine system in pathology of pet and aviary birds. Ames (IA): Blackwell/Iowa State Press; 2003.

[39] Bachman SE, Mashaly MM. Relationship between circulating thyroid hormones and humoral immunity in immature male chickens. Dev Comp Immunol 1986;10:395–403.

[40] Sundlick RS, herdegen D, Brown TR, et al. Thyroidal iodine metabolism in obese-strain chickens before immune mediated challenge. J Endocrinol 1991;128:239–44.

[41] Dietrich HM, Oliveira dos Santos AJ, Wick G. Development of spontaneous autoimmune thyroiditis in obese strain [OS] chickens. Vet Immunol Immunopathol 1997;57:141–6.

[42] Wick G, Andersson L, Hala K, et al. Avian models with spontaneous autoimmune diseases. Adv Immunol 2006;92:71–117.

[43] Schmidt RE. Immune system. In: Altman RB, Clubb SL, Dorrestein GM, et al, editors. Avian medicine and surgery. Philadelphia: Saunders; 1997. p. 645–52.

[44] Rae M. Endocrine disease in pet birds. Sem Avian Exotic Pet Med 1995;4:32–8.

[45] Schmidt RE, Reavill DR. Thyroid hyperplasia in birds. J Avian Med Surg 2002;16:111–4.

[46] Wadsworth PF, Jones DM. Some abnormalities of the thyroid gland in non-domesticated birds. Avian Pathol 1979;8:279–84.

[47] Ivanics E, Rudas P, Salye G, et al. Massive goitre [struma parenchymatosa] in geese. Acta Vet Hung 1999;47:217–31.

[48] Merryman JI, Buckles EL. The avian thyroid gland. Part two: a review of function and pathophysiology. J Avian Med Surg 1998;12:238–42.

[49] Oglesbee B. Hypothyroidism in a scarlet macaw. J Am Vet Med Assoc 1992;201:1599–601.

[50] Otsuka R, Aoki K, Hori H, et al. Changes in circulating LH, sex steroid hormones, thyroid hormones and corticosterone in relation to breeding and molting in captive humboldt penguins [*Spheniscus humboldti*] kept in an outdoor open display. Zoolog Sci 1998;15:103–9.

[51] Pant K, Chandola-Saklani A. Effects of thyroxine on avian moulting may not involve prior conversion to triiodothyronine. J Endocrinol 1993;137:265–70.

[52] Szelenyi Z, Peczely P. Thyroxin induced moult in domestic hen. Acta Physiol Hung 1988;72:143–9.

[53] King AS, McLelland J. Endocrine system in birds: their structure and function. London: Bailliere Tindall; 1985.

[54] Harms CA, Hoskinson JJ, Bruyette DS, et al. Development of an experimental model of hypothyroidism in cockatiels [*Nymphicus hollandicus*]. Am J Vet Res 1994;55:399–404.

[55] Leach MW. A survey of neoplasia in pet birds. Sem Avian Exotic Pet Med 1992;1:52–64.

[56] Bates G, Tucker RL, Ford S, et al. Thyroid adenocarcinoma in a bald eagle [*Haliaeetus leukocephalus*]. J Zoo Wildl Med 1999;30:439–42.

[57] Schmidt RE. Morphologic diagnosis of avian neoplasms. Sem Avian Exotic Pet Med 1992;1:73–9.

ELSEVIER
SAUNDERS

Vet Clin Exot Anim 11 (2008) 25–34

VETERINARY
CLINICS
Exotic Animal Practice

The Avian Pancreas in Health and Disease

Anthony A. Pilny, DVM, DABVP–Avian

Avian and Exotic Pet Medicine, Lenox Hill Veterinarians, 204 East 76th Street,
New York, NY 10021, USA

The avian pancreas lies suspended between the ascending and descending duodenum, conveniently located to contribute its hormonal mix to the portal vein that has been recently loaded with absorbed nutrients [1]. In most birds it is composed of three lobes: dorsal, ventral, and splenic with the dorsal and ventral lobes remaining separate in the pigeon and duck. The endocrine portion of the avian pancreas (focus of this article) occupies considerably more tissue mass than in mammals and the distribution of cell types differs as well. There are three types of islets described, which vary according to lobar location and species. The dark islets are composed mostly of A cells with some D cells and the light islets contain a mixture of B and D cells. The third type, the mixed islets, has all three cell types: A, B, and D cells. The dark islets are irregularly shaped, large, and indistinctly separated from the exocrine pancreatic tissue. The light islets by contrast are round to elliptical in shape, compact, and distinct from the exocrine tissue [2]. A cells synthesize and release glucagon; B cells synthesize and release insulin; D cells secrete somatostatin. The exocrine pancreas supplies digestive juice through ducts to aid in small intestinal digestion. A fourth cell type of the avian pancreas, the F cell, sometimes called the PP cell, makes and releases pancreatic polypeptide or APP. It should be recognized that most of our knowledge of the avian endocrine pancreas originates from experimental work with domestic granivorous species [3–8].

Avian insulin is a powerful anabolic hormone and is many times more potent than mammalian insulin in stimulating glycogenesis and hypoglycemia [1]. Glucagon is a powerful catabolic hormone in birds and circulates at levels up to eight times higher than humans [1]. Increases in blood glucose will stimulate pancreatic B-cell activity, triggering release of insulin, and decreasing blood glucose levels will elicit the release of glucagon. Absorbed

E-mail address: apilny@avianexoticpetvet.com

nutrients will stimulate D-cell activity as does A-cell activity. By sharing the same extracellular fluid with the islet, paracrine modulation of endocrine secretion takes place in the avian pancreas. The A cell stimulates both B- and D-cell activity and closes the negative feedback. The D cell most likely regulates the proportion of insulin (I) secreted to glucagon (G) secreted at the same time, adjusting the I/G molar ratio to meet the individual's needs at that time [9]. Pancreatic polypeptide, the product of the F cell, circulates at levels up to 40 times higher than in humans. It functions to inhibit gastrointestinal motility and secretion as well as exocrine pancreatic secretion.

Carbohydrate metabolism differs significantly in birds compared with mammals. The fasting blood glucose level of most birds ranges from 150% to 300% above fasted mammals. How birds can survive with blood glucose levels that would be consistent with uncontrolled diabetes in mammals is unknown. Important differences between birds and mammals include, first, that embryonic birds develop in a very different metabolic environment protected within the egg with a yolk sac rather than placental attachment to a mother with shared circulating nutrients. Second, current evidence shows that glucagon is the dominant hormone regulating carbohydrate metabolism in birds, whereas insulin is considered to be the dominant pancreatic hormone in mammals [9]. This does not mean insulin should be ignored because anti-insulin antibodies will induce a long-lasting hyperglycemia in ducks [10]. Last, fasting glucose metabolism in birds is approximately twice that of fasted mammals.

B-cell release of insulin in birds is basically similar to mammals with a few notable exceptions. Glucose is not a trigger for insulin release with the B cell being more responsive to glucagon, cholecystokinin, and absorbed amino acids. Specifically, a synergism exists between glucose and amino acids in regulating insulin secretion and epinephrine, secretin, and fatty acids do not appear to affect insulin release in birds. To sum up, the release of insulin from the avian islet is the result of numerous inputs, namely endocrine, exocrine, paracrine, neural, and humoral. Short-term fasting has little effect on circulating levels of insulin in chickens and ducks.

A-cell release of glucagon is triggered by free fatty acids and cholecystokinin. Glucose has an inhibitory effect on glucagon release from the avian A cell. Glucagon receptors appear in much greater numbers than insulin receptors in a given tissue, supporting the suggestion that glucagon is the dominant hormone of avian carbohydrate metabolism [9].

Somatostatin concentration in the avian pancreas can range up to 150 times greater than the mammalian pancreas and its function appears to be identical in suppressing islet hormone release, slowing nutrient absorption, and modifying the I/G ratio. Release of this hormone is by neural, hormonal, humoral, and paracrine control. The role of this hormone in suppressing the activity of neighboring pancreatic islet cells and adjusting the I/G molar ratio prepares the bird for either a catabolic or anabolic state as the metabolic need dictates. Normal I/G molar ratios in birds are generally half those of mammals [9]. The ratio, therefore, maintains a catabolic state in birds ensuring plentiful fuel supply to meet a high rate of metabolism for stressful conditions such as egg laying, fasting, and sustained migratory flight.

Surgical pancreatectomy

Experiments involving removal of the avian pancreas date back to the late 1800s. These early studies not only helped to identify the pancreas as the organ controlling mammalian carbohydrate metabolism, but also led to the belief that birds would not become permanent diabetics after surgical removal of the pancreas. Newer studies have shown the opposite is true in that complete removal of the pancreas will lead to a severe hypoglycemic crisis requiring repeated glucagon and/or glucose infusions to prevent moribund seizures [5]. Glucose is essential to life, especially during periods of fasting. Other studies have shown that anti-insulin antibodies cause hyperglycemia in depancreatized ducks indicating that insulin is also necessary for glucoregulation [10]. An additional observation is that a secondary source of insulin may exist in birds since there is a persistence of circulating insulin for up to 10 days after surgery [1]. Subtotal pancreatectomy results in a transient diabetic state in ducks with a return to normal blood glucose levels in 2 weeks. In geese, a permanent diabetic state is attained [6]. The maintenance of normal responsiveness to glucose by the avian islet A cell requires the presence of insulin. In summary, the most significant finding is that glucagon is important to birds for normal glucoregulation, and that insulin is needed for complete normalcy. Last, glucagon is more important in the fasted bird and insulin is more important in the fed bird.

Altered metabolism

Diabetes mellitus is the most recognized disease of the pancreas owing to its prevalence in human and feline patients. The clinical condition seen in birds is controversial because of the differences between mammals and birds and because the exact pathogenesis is unclear in birds. Historically, many cases of diabetes, or hyperglycemia without ketonuria, have been attributed to another primary disease such as disorders of the liver, stress, or reproductive diseases (eg, yolk coelomitis/peritonitis), although primary diabetes mellitus appears to be more commonly diagnosed as a clinical syndrome in pet birds. Additional factors, such as peripheral insulin resistance and exogenous or endogenous glucocorticoids, may contribute to hyperglycemia in companion birds as well. Some believe that insulin may not be as important for glucose regulation in granivorous birds as it is for mammals, and that diabetes mellitus in granivorous birds may not be caused by insulin abnormalities at all, although newer articles are showing that primary diabetes does occur in birds [11].

Primary diabetes mellitus has been reported and described in budgerigars (*Melopsittacus undulates*) [12–14], Toco toucans (*Ramphastos toco*) [15,16], an African gray parrot (*Psittacus erithacus*) [17], Chestnut-fronted macaw (*Ara severa*) [18], and a Red-tailed hawk (*Buteo jamaicensis*) [19]. Other case reports have described diabetes mellitus in a cockatiel (*Nymphicus hollandicus*), a Hyacinth macaw (*Anodorhynchus hyacinthinus*), an Emperor penguin (*Aptenodytes forsteri*), and a Military macaw (*Ara militaris*) [20–22]. In these cases, diabetes was diagnosed or suspected by findings of either hyperglycemia or glucosuria, although not all birds had pancreatic lesions. Information in the peer-reviewed literature regarding diabetes mellitus in pet birds is scarce with most being case reports consisting of small numbers of birds as referenced above.

Etiology

In humans and domestic mammals, gross or microscopic changes to pancreatic islet cells are rarely of value in diagnosing diabetes mellitus. The reported range of lesions that may be associated with type 1 diabetes (insulin-dependent) include a reduced number and size of pancreatic islets and pancreatitis. Both of these lesions reflect the postulated hypotheses that type 1 diabetes is a result of genetic, environmental, or autoimmune factors that reduce the overall functional mass of pancreatic B cells [18].

Type 2 (non–insulin dependent) diabetes mellitus, the most common form in people, is characterized by insulin resistance, lack of insulin production from the β-cells, and inappropriate hepatic glucose secretion. Type 2 diabetes primarily has been associated with the β-cell production and progressive deposition of islet amyloid polypeptide (IAPP), mainly in humans and cats. It is not yet clear what role IAPP plays in the pathogenesis of diabetes mellitus, especially in regard to whether deposition of IAPP is a cause of or a response to diabetes mellitus. However, the absence of islet (insular) amyloidosis does not necessarily preclude a diagnosis of diabetes mellitus. Conversely, the presence of islet amyloidosis does not always translate into clinical diabetes mellitus. At this time, islet amyloidosis has not been reported in avian species, which may suggest that either type 2 diabetes does not occur in birds or its prevalence is so low that clinical detection is rare [18].

Mirsky and colleagues [10] reported that diabetes mellitus can be induced in ducks by administration of anti-insulin antibodies. Gancz and colleagues [22] recently proposed that diabetes mellitus may be associated with iron-storage disease (hepatic hemosiderosis in this article) in psittacine birds without pancreatic inflammatory lesions.

Signalment

A specific signalment cannot be stated. Published case reports generally include a single patient or small number of cases and vary in age and species.

Currently, there are no studies to determine if any age, sex, hereditary factors, or species predilection in birds exists.

History

Diabetes mellitus should be considered a differential diagnosis for the avian patient presenting with classic signs of polyuria, polydipsia, weight loss, and polyphagia. In some cases and in those with concurrent disease, nonspecific signs such as depression, regurgitation, or anorexia may be seen. It is important to distinguish diarrhea from polyuria when evaluating the avian patient. Polyuria is an increase in urine volume and clients often complain of the cage paper becoming soaked rapidly. Diarrhea is increased fluid in the fecal portion and the feces will not be formed or easily identified from the urine and urates portion in bird droppings (Fig. 1).

Physical examination

Physical examination of the diabetic patient may reveal no abnormalities or show decreased pectoral muscle mass and loss of body fat. Increased eyelid turgor and dry mucus membranes can indicate dehydration despite severe polydipsia. Birds may be weak, depressed, and prefer to stay at the bottom of the cage too weak to perch. Polyuria is evident in most cases.

Diagnosis

The normal range for plasma glucose in pet birds is significantly higher than that observed in mammals, with ranges from 180 to 350 mg/dL,

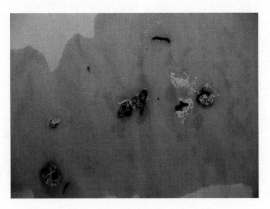

Fig. 1. Polyuria and polydipsia in a pet bird. Note the increased amounts of urine soaking the cage paper and formed feces differentiating diarrhea from polyuria.

depending on the species. One should be cautious not to base the diagnosis of diabetes mellitus on fasting glucose concentration alone since many birds may develop a transient hyperglycemia when stressed. Fasted blood glucose levels above 800 mg/dL are diagnostic and most birds present with values well above 1000 mg/dL. Blood glucose concentrations this high will surpass the renal threshold and glucose will spill into the urine making urine dip strips useful in smaller patients (or with daily insulin management) (Fig. 2). Performing a urinalysis in birds may be difficult since the urine is mixed with the feces and urates in the cloaca before passing, thus altering results. When possible, and in most polyuric birds, the liquid portion of the dropping should be aspirated with a syringe or nonheparinized capillary tube carefully avoiding fecal contamination, which may falsely elevate glucose readings. Normal avian urine is reported to be "negative" on the glucose reagent strip. The finding of ketonuria in birds is abnormal and is strongly supportive of diabetes when hyperglycemia and glucosuria are present. A thorough diagnostic medical workup including complete blood count, biochemical profile, survey radiographs, viral screening, and other patient-specific testing is necessary to rule out other diseases that may be causes of hyperglycemia. It is often recommended to obtain a pancreatic biopsy in avian patients for definitive diagnosis; however, this is not common practice in the medical workup of any other species with these clinical signs and may be too risky. Schmidt and Reavill [23] reported nonspecific

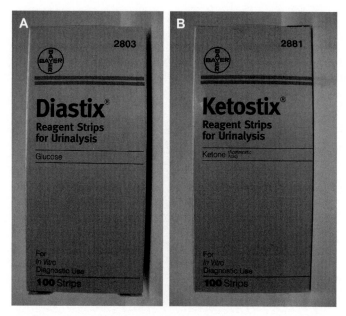

Fig. 2. Urine glucose (A) and ketone strips (B) should be used in birds with polyuria and polydipsia.

degeneration of pancreatic islet cells was the most common condition seen in pancreatic necropsy specimens taking the form of vacuolation of islet cells with variable cellular loss. Some of these cases had been associated with clinical diabetes mellitus, but clinical signs were nonspecific or absent in many. The significance of fructosamine concentrations in birds is unknown at this time but may be useful in diabetic management of avian patients [22]. The use of immunohistochemistry of the avian pancreas has been reported with success although this test is not clinically readily available [18,24].

Treatment

The small number of existing clinical reports support that diabetic birds can respond to insulin therapy [2,15,20,22,25], although one macaw had no response despite increased dosing (Fig. 3) [18]. In the author's experience, birds that have profound or abnormal responses to insulin most likely are not primary diabetics but have a different underlying cause for the hyperglycemia. Two cases that illustrate this are a hyperglycemic cockatiel diagnosed with severe hepatic fibrosis and a hyperglycemic sun conure diagnosed with pancreatic adenocarcinoma where both birds showed classic clinical signs of diabetes. Both birds became severely hypoglycemic within an hour of the lowest dose of insulin administered requiring life-saving treatment.

Birds that are depressed, dehydrated, anoretic, and/or vomiting require appropriate fluid therapy and nutritional support. Treatment of any underlying disorder is necessary for the successful management of diabetes mellitus. Birds should be hospitalized when insulin therapy is begun when attempting to regulate the patient. A serial blood glucose curve should be performed when possible, measuring blood glucose concentrations before insulin administration and then every 2 to 3 hours for up to 24 hours. This is especially important in birds, since the response to insulin therapy

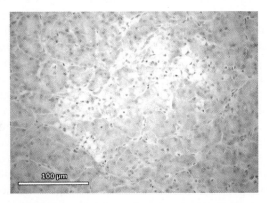

Fig. 3. Immunohistochemical staining of the pancreas of a diabetic macaw showing vaculated islet cells are negative for insulin (immunohistochemical stain, ×400).

can be erratic and vary with species or individuals due in part to insulin resistance and the development of pancreatic insufficiency and pancreatic atrophy. Furthermore, the peak and duration of effect of insulin preparations currently available are unknown in avian species. The glucose blood curve will aid in determining a proper dose of insulin for the patient. Gancz and colleagues [22] reported that bovine and porcine protamine-zinc insulin produced the best long-term control of clinical signs. These authors also reported that use of glipizide and human recombinant insulin produced little or no response in a previously published conference proceedings paper [26].

In the hospitalized patient, initial therapy with regular insulin at subcutaneous or intramuscular (IM) doses of 0.1 to 0.2 U/kg is instituted. Plasma glucose concentrations are monitored every 2 to 3 hours depending on the patient, and the dosage is adjusted until blood glucose concentration is maintained closer to the normal range. Urine reagent strips are used frequently in smaller birds where repeated blood sampling is not possible. When the bird is stable, therapy with longer-acting insulin is begun. Birds with uncomplicated diabetes not requiring hospitalization are immediately begun on neutral protamine Hagedorn or protamine zinc insulin, but should likewise be hospitalized for a serial blood glucose curve, adjusting the insulin dosage until blood glucose concentration is maintained within an acceptable range. Dosages will vary significantly between birds, and should be individually titrated. An extremely wide range of dosages have been reported (from 0.002 IU/bird to 3.0 IU/kg IM every 12 to 48 hours), most of which are extrapolated from mammalian dosages [27]. Insulin may be and is often diluted with sterile water for accurate dosing and will remain stable under refrigeration for 30 days. Use of newer insulin glargine preparations, such as Lantus (sanofi-aventis US LLC, Bridgewater, NJ), may prove useful in avian patients but use is anecdotal at this time.

Once an initial dosage of insulin has been determined, the bird is sent home on insulin injections, to be administered by the owner providing the owner is comfortable and capable. In most cases, twice daily injections are necessary although some birds may only require insulin every few days. The goals of long-term home management are to eliminate weight loss and reduce the clinical signs of polyphagia, polyuria, and polydypsia. The value of strict control of hyperglycemia must be weighed against the possibility of inducing hypoglycemia, which could be life threatening. If the urine is used to monitor insulin therapy at home, it is usually necessary to maintain a slight hyperglycemia and subsequent polyuria to obtain a urine sample to test. The urine is monitored with test reagent strips two times daily or whenever a viable sample is available. Urine glucose should be maintained at slight positive or "trace," and the insulin dosage adjusted accordingly. It is important to advise the owner of signs of hypoglycemia, such as extreme lethargy, weakness, and seizures and possible home treatment until the bird can be evaluated and treated in the hospital. The bird should return to the hospital for serial blood glucose monitoring 1 week after the initiation of insulin therapy, since it is likely that several days are required for glucose homeostasis to equilibrate (as is the case in mammals). The serial blood glucose curve should also be reevaluated whenever clinical signs of diabetes and glycosuria become persistent, or every 6 months in the well-controlled bird.

Oral hypoglycemic medication

Glipizide (Glucotrol, Pfizer Inc, New York, NY) has been used in the management of diabetic birds with varied to no success as seen by the author. Glipizide is commonly used in the treatment of Type 2 diabetes in humans and cats. The primary effect of this sulfonylurea class drug is to stimulate insulin production and release by pancreatic beta cells. Other possible effects include inhibition of hepatic gluconeogenesis and increased peripheral insulin sensitivity. As with insulin therapy, the goal of treatment is to decrease the clinical signs of hyperglycemia; not to achieve tight regulation of serum glucose concentration. The reported dose for birds is 0.5 mg/kg twice daily [21]. Another option is to dissolve a 10 mg tablet in the bird's drinking water daily and allow the bird to self-medicate because of the polydipsia. There are no reports of use of other oral hypoglycemic drugs in birds at this time.

Dietary modification

As with diabetic mammals, a high-fiber diet should be fed. Appropriate modifications to existing diets should be made after recovery and slowly to ensure the patient is on an appropriate diet.

Summary

The lack of knowledge of the pathophysiologic mechanism of diabetes mellitus in pet birds makes management of this condition difficult. It requires long-term monitoring and flexibility on the part of the veterinarian and pet bird owner. Therapy should be based on current knowledge and appropriate extrapolation of treatment of mammalian species. Understanding the physiology of the avian pancreas will allow for better treatment by the clinician.

References

[1] Hazelwood RL. Pancreas. In: Whittow GC, editor. Sturkie's avian physiology. 5th edition. San Diego: Academic Press; 2000. p. 539–55.
[2] Oglesbee BL, Orosz S, Dorrestein GM. The endocrine system. In: Altman RB, Clubb SL, Dorrestein GM, editors. Avian medicine and surgery. Philadelphia: WB Saunders; 1997. p. 475–88.

[3] Karmann H, Mialhe P. Glucose, insulin and glucagon in the diabetic goose. Horm Metab Res 1976;8:419–26.

[4] Laurent F, Mialhe P. Insulin and the glucose-glucagon feedback mechanism in the duck. Diabetologia 1976;12:23–33.

[5] Laurent F, Gross R, Lakili M, et al. Effect of insulin on glucagon secretion mediated via glucose metabolism of pancreatic A cells in ducks. Diabetologia 1981;20:72–7.

[6] Karmann H, Mialhe P. Progressive loss of sensitivity of the A cell to insulin in geese made diabetic by subtotal pancreatectomy. Horm Metab Res 1982;14:452–8.

[7] Laurent F, Mialhe A, Boulanger Y, et al. Amino acids in normal and diabetic ducks. Horm Metab Res 1985;17:223–5.

[8] Laurent F, Karmann H, Gross R, et al. Glucagon and somatostatin secretion from the perfused splenic bulb of duck pancreas. Acta Endocrinol (Copenh) 1986;113:272–80.

[9] Hazelwood RL. Pancreatic hormones, insulin/glucagon molar ratios, and somatostatin as determinants of avian carbohydrate metabolism. J Exp Zool 1984;232(3):647–52.

[10] Mirsky IA, Jinks R, Perisutti G. Production of diabetes mellitus in the duck by insulin antibodies. Am J Physiol 1964;206:133–5.

[11] Rae M. Avian endocrine disorders. In: Fudge AM, editor. Laboratory medicine. Avian and exotic pets. Philadelphia: WB Saunders; 2000. p. 76–98.

[12] Appleby RC. Diabetes mellitus in a budgerigar (Melopsittacus undulates). Vet Rec 1984; 115(25–26):652–3.

[13] Altman RB, Kirmayer AH. Diabetes mellitus in the avian species. J Am Anim Hosp Assoc 1976;12:531–7.

[14] Ryan CP, Walder EJ, Howard EB. Diabetes mellitus and islet cell carcinoma in a parakeet. J Am Anim Hosp Assoc 1982;18:139–42.

[15] Douglass EM. Diabetes mellitus in a toco toucan. Mod Vet Pract 1981;62:293–5.

[16] Murphy J. Diabetes in toucans. Proc Annu Conf Assoc Avian Vet 1992;165–70.

[17] Candeletta SC, Homer BL, Harner MM, et al. Diabetes mellitus associated with chronic lymphocytic pancreatitis in an African Grey Parrot (Psittacus erithacus erithacus). J Assoc Avian Vet 1993;7(1):39–43.

[18] Pilny AA, Luong R. Diabetes mellitus in a chestnut-fronted macaw. J Avian Med Surg 2005; 19(4):297–302.

[19] Wallner-Pendleton EA, Rogers D, Epple A. Diabetes mellitus in a red-tailed hawk. Avian Pathol 1993;22:631–5.

[20] Bonda M. Plasma glucagon, serum insulin, and serum amylase levels in normal and hyperglycemic macaw. Proc Annu Conf Assoc Avian Vet 1996;77–88.

[21] Pollock CG, Pledger T. Diabetes mellitus in avian species. Proc Annu Conf Assoc Avian Vet 2001;151–4.

[22] Gancz AY, Wellehan JF, Boutette J, et al. Diabetes mellitus concurrent with hepatic haemosiderosis in two macaws (Ara severa, Ara militaris). Avian Pathol 2007;36(4):331–6.

[23] Schmidt RE, Reavill DR. Endocrine lesions in psittacine birds. Proc Annu Conf Assoc Avian Vet 2006;27–9.

[24] Gulmez N, Kocamis H, Aslan A, et al. Immunohistochemical distribution of cells containing insulin, glucagon, and somatostatin in the goose (Anser anser) pancreas. Turk J Vet Anim Sci 2004;28:403–7.

[25] Lumeij JT. Endocrinology. In: Ritchie BW, Harrison GJ, Harrison LR, editors. Avian medicine: principles and application. Lake Worth (FL): HBD International Inc.; 1999. p. 582–606.

[26] Gancz AY, Wellehan JF, Boutette J, et al. Diabetes mellitus in large psittacines: a possible relationship with excessive iron storage. Proc Annu Conf Assoc Avian Vet 2005;267–9.

[27] Carpenter JW. Exotic animal formulary. 3rd edition. St. Louis: Elsevier; 2005. p. 214.

VETERINARY
CLINICS
Exotic Animal Practice

ELSEVIER
SAUNDERS

Vet Clin Exot Anim 11 (2008) 35–57

Adrenal Steroid Metabolism in Birds: Anatomy, Physiology, and Clinical Considerations

Ricardo de Matos, LMV, DABVP–Avian

Section of Wildlife and Exotic Medicine, Department of Clinical Sciences,
College of Veterinary Medicine, Cornell University, Ithaca, NY 14853-6401, USA

Steroid hormones in mammals can be grouped into five categories according to the receptors to which they bind: glucocorticoids, mineralocorticoids, androgens, estrogens, and progestagens. The natural steroid hormones are generally synthesized from cholesterol in the gonads and adrenal glands (Fig. 1). Corticosteroids (glucocorticoids and mineralocorticoids) are a class of steroid hormones that are produced in the adrenal cortex. They are involved in a wide range of physiologic systems such as stress response, immune response and regulation of inflammation, carbohydrate metabolism, protein catabolism, blood electrolyte levels, and behavior. The hypothalamo-pituitary-adrenal (HPA) axis mediates secretion and release of corticosteroids from the adrenal gland. The HPA system in birds is anatomically and functionally different from mammals, with corticosterone being the main glucocorticoid and aldosterone being produced only in small amounts. As a result of this, the response of birds to endogenous and exogenous corticosteroids is likely different from the response in mammals [1].

Adrenal gland anatomy

The right and left adrenal glands are small, yellowish, ovoid glands, located craniomedial to the kidneys and gonads [1,2]. They lie close together and may be fused in some species (rhea) [2]. In many species, the male bird may have an appendix epididymis that extends from the epididymis into the adrenal gland, or adrenal tissue may be found within the epididymis [2].

E-mail address: rd95@cornell.edu

1094-9194/08/$ - see front matter © 2008 Elsevier Inc. All rights reserved.
doi:10.1016/j.cvex.2007.09.006
vetexotic.theclinics.com

Major biosynthetic pathways of steroid hormone production.

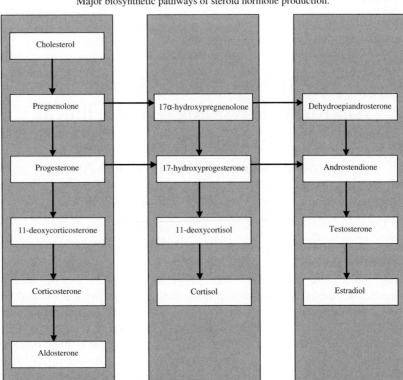

Fig. 1. Major biosynthetic pathways of steroid hormone production.

Blood supply to the glands is through the cranial renal arteries and occasionally directly from the aorta. Each gland has a single adrenal vein that
drains into the caudal vena cava [1]. An adrenal portal system between
each gland and the abdominal wall musculature may also occur [2]. In
addition, in the chicken, each gland receives one or two lymphatic vessels.
Preganglionic sympathetic fibers from the thoracic and synsacral splanchnic
nerves converge on the cranial and caudal ganglia located in the fibrous capsule of the gland or embedded in the gland tissue. Unmyelinated postganglionic fibers synapse with a number of chromaffin cells found in the medulla
[1].

The avian adrenal parenchyma is composed of an intermingling of
adrenocortical and chromaffin tissue, without the distinct histologic regions
of outer cortex and inner medulla found in the adrenals of mammals.
Adrenocortical and chromaffin tissues constitute about 58% and 42% of
the parenchyma respectively [1].

Adrenocortical cells are arranged in cords composed of a double row of cells that radiate from the center of the gland and loop against the inner surface of the connective tissue capsule. The arrangement of specific cell types along the cords results in some structural and functional zonation with formation of two regions: a subcapsular zone, reminiscent of mammalian zona glomerulosa cells, and a more extensive inner zone, reminiscent of mammalian zona fasciculata/reticularis. This zonation is apparent in the duck, chicken, and brown pelican and is most distinct when corticotrophic stimulation is suppressed or enhanced. Subcapsular zone cells produce larger amounts of aldosterone than corticosterone in response to pituitary adrenocorticotrophic hormone (ACTH), and produce aldosterone exclusively in response to angiotensin II. In contrast, the inner zone cells produce larger amounts of corticosterone than aldosterone in response to ACTH [1]. The inner zone cells are also more sensitive and more responsive to ACTH stimulation than are the cells of the subcapsular zone [3].

Chromaffin cells are more concentrated centrally in the gland and gather in clusters, each innervated by a single nerve bundle, as in mammals. The avian adrenal gland has two types of chromaffin cells: those releasing epinephrine and those releasing norepinephrine, with the proportions of each cell type varying with species [1].

Adrenocortical physiology

Adrenocortical hormones

The major function of the avian adrenocortical cells is to produce glucocorticoid and mineralocorticoid hormones, with corticosterone being the most important corticoid hormone produced in adult birds [1,4]. This is in contrast to the mammalian adrenal gland, which secretes approximately three to four times more cortisol than corticosterone [4]. The mineralocorticoid aldosterone is produced in considerably less quantity in birds. The average ratio of basal circulating aldosterone to corticosterone is around 1:100 in mature birds. During the embryonic and perinatal periods, the avian adrenal gland also synthesizes significant quantities of other corticosteroids, including cortisol and cortisone, and sex steroids, such as testosterone and estradiol [1,5]. In the embryonic stage, the adrenal gland is a more important source of testosterone than either the ovary or testes [5]. The production of these additional steroids by the avian adrenal gland declines rapidly after hatching [5,6]; however, measurable concentrations of plasma cortisol have been reported in some adult species of psittacines [7–9] and in condors (*Vulture* gryphus) [10].

Corticosteroid hormones are biosynthesized from cholesterol following similar pathways that have been described in mammals (see Fig. 1), mostly involving cytochrome P-450 enzymes [1,11].

Corticosterone in birds is transported in the blood bound to two specific plasma proteins: transcortin or corticosteroid binding globulin (CBG), a specific binding protein with high affinity and low binding capacity, and albumin, which has a low affinity and nonspecific high binding capacity [1,2,5]. The concentration of these transport proteins is influenced by a variety of factors, such as thyroxin, testosterone, and hypophysectomy, all three decreasing CBG concentration [2]. The level of circulating corticosterone is controlled in part by its binding to these proteins, since, when bound, corticosterone availability to target cells is reduced and renal and hepatic clearance limited [1,2]. Despite this, glucocorticoid target cells appear to be able to selectively bind to and cleave CBG to enhance steroid bioavailability/activity. Different tissues may express different levels of steroid-binding proteins, which would explain the differences in steroid activity among these tissues. Also, the variation in expression of the different CBG isoforms with different specificities/affinities for cortisol, corticosterone and other glucocorticoid metabolites could explain the shifting pattern of glucocorticoid metabolite secretion by the adrenal gland during developmental, neonatal, and maturation phases [1].

The blood concentrations of corticosteroids are maintained by the dynamic balance of adrenal secretion and metabolic clearance by the liver and kidney. The half-life of corticosterone and aldosterone in avian species is about 15 minutes. The metabolic clearance rate for corticosterone varies with physiological status, decreasing with age and increasing with dietary protein restriction [1].

Regulation of adrenocortical hormone production

The secretion of corticosterone, and probably aldosterone, is mediated primarily by the hypothalamus-pituitary-adrenal (HPA) axis by pituitary adrenocorticotrophic hormone (ACTH). Corticotropin-releasing factor (CRF) produced by the hypothalamus stimulates the release of ACTH from the pituitary in response to stress [1,6]. Peak plasma ACTH levels are achieved within 5 to 10 minutes after the stimulus, with ACTH inducing a rapid and dose-dependent release of corticosterone and, to a lesser degree, aldosterone. Arginine vasotocin (AVT) also stimulates ACTH secretion in some avian species. The relative response of avian pituitary gland to CRF and AVT change with different physiological and ecological conditions. Glucocorticoids exert a negative feedback at all levels of the HPA axis decreasing the release of ACTH. ACTH release from the pituitary is also inhibited by somatostatin and opioids [1].

The regulation of aldosterone secretion in birds is likely similar to mammals. Renin is released from the juxtaglomerular cells of the kidney in response to low plasma sodium concentration or reduced blood volume [1,6]. In contrast to mammals, hyperkalemia does not activate the renin-angiotensin system (RAS) in birds [6]. Renin converts circulating angiotensinogen to angiotensin I, which is then converted to angiotensin II. Angiotensin II stimulates the adrenal gland directly to release aldosterone and also corticosterone, rather than by stimulating the release of ACTH from the pituitary [1,2,6]. ACTH can also stimulate the release of aldosterone, although the release of the ACTH does not appear to be induced by changes in the electrolyte and hemodynamic balance. In many anseriform species, changes in the RAS and the HPA axis are integrated to influence the overall stress response. The RAS role in controlling aldosterone secretion in birds is less precise and important than in mammals. This, in part, may be because of the lack of a distinct organization of the adrenal steroidogenic tissue. RAS importance in birds varies between species according to their natural habitat and food sources [1]. Angiotensin II has been shown to be a potent dipsogen in a variety of birds, with a marked correlation between blood levels and pattern of water intake in quail. On the other side, carnivorous birds (that ingest most of the water requirements with food) and xerophilous birds, such as the budgerigar (with low water requirements) show a much lower sensitivity to angiotensinogen II [6].

Although ACTH is the most efficacious stimulator of avian corticosteroid secretion, many other secretory products of the peripheral immune, neural, and endocrine organs and other circulating factors can stimulate or modulate adrenocortical function and its response to stress. They can act as stimulator/positive modulator or as inhibitor/negative modulator, with some being able to do both depending on other factors. Table 1 summarizes modulators of adrenocortical function.

Despite changes associated with stress, blood concentrations of corticosteroids follow patterns according to variations in physiological and ecological contexts, mainly photoperiod, reproductive status, season, and age [1].

Table 1
Modulators of adrenocortical function [1,5,12]

Stimulator/positive modulator	Inhibitor/negative modulator	Biphasic modulator
ACTH (pituitary and activated lymphocytes)	Glucocorticoids	T3 (inhibitor with protein restriction)
Angiotensin II	Vagal tone	Prostaglandins
Prolactin	Acetylcholine	Gonadal steroids
Growth hormone	Bursal antisteroidogenic peptide	Catecholamine
Parathyroid hormone (mainly A)	Somatostatin (via ACTH)	
Serotonin	Opioids (via ACTH)	
Vasoactive intestinal peptide		
Interleukin-1 (activated immune cells)		
Bursa of Fabricious secretory product		
Melatonin		
Opioids		
Arginine vasotocin (via ACTH)		
Corticotropin-releasing factor (via ACTH)		
Mesotocin		
Insulin		

Abbreviations: A, aldosterone; ACTH, adrenocorticotrophic hormone; C corticosterone.

Studies in Japanese quail, pigeons, chickens, turkeys, and ducks have shown a distinct daily pattern of circulating corticosterone blood concentrations [1]. In general, maximum concentrations are found during the night or at the transition of the dark-light phases [1,5,11]. The variation of corticosterone concentration with the circadian rhythm is thought to provide energy in homeothermic animals during nocturnal periods, when not feeding or moving. For nocturnal species, such as owls, circulating corticosterone concentrations may be more correlated with activity period than light-dark cycle. This daily variation in corticosterone concentration in birds results from changes in secretion of CRF and ACTH, sensitivity of the adrenal gland to ACTH and stress, corticosterone secretion rate, and corticosterone clearance rate. The hypothalamus is considered the pacemaker that controls variation in corticosterone concentration with circadian rhythm. The suprachiasmic nucleus of the hypothalamus receives information from the retina and pineal gland and melatonin is the effector substance, both at the HPA axis and adrenal gland levels [1].

Seasonal changes, which reflect changes in the photoperiod, temperature, and food availability, can also cause seasonal variation in adrenocortical activity, with activity being greatest in mid-winter and least in the summer [5]. This variation helps birds adapt to physiologic changes, such as altered reproductive status, migration, and molting, and to environmental changes, including limited food availability and territoriality [1].

There is also variation of corticosterone concentration associated with reproductive status, with higher levels noted during the breeding season. This variation is a result of enhanced adrenocortical response to ACTH and reduced glucocorticoid negative feedback on the HPA axis during this time period. During the nonbreeding periods of normal molt and migration, the regression of the reproductive system is associated with decreased adrenocortical function and decreased levels of corticosterone. Exception to this is the food/water-deprivation–induced molt in the domestic hen, in which regression of the reproductive system is associated with an increase in circulating corticosterone secondary to food restriction [1].

Adrenocortical activity also changes with age, gradually declining after hatching until birds reach sexual maturity. This change is characterized by decreased secretion rates (and metabolic clearance rates) of corticosterone, and decreased resting and stress-induced and ACTH-induced plasma corticosterone concentrations, possibly from decreased adrenocortical sensitivity to ACTH [1].

Physiological effects of adrenocortical hormones

Adrenal corticosteroids influence the metabolic processes of almost every cell in the body and produce diverse effects. They exert their effects after binding to specific nuclear receptors, which have been found in avian brain, liver, kidney, lung, intestine, muscle, thymus, bursa of Fabricius, and nasal gland [1,11]. Corticosteroids may act directly on target tissues or, as described above, their effects may be modulated by interactions with other hormones, including thyroid hormone, growth hormone, prolactin, norepinephrine, and somatomedin C [1]. Corticosteroids play a major role in the maintenance of homeostasis, cardiac and skeletal muscle strength, brain activity, electrolyte regulation, and water compartment distribution, together with managing the organism's response to stress [1,6,11]. A stressor is defined as any biochemical, sensory, visual, or emotional stimulus of sufficient intensity that requires major adjustments in or are threats to homeostasis [1]. These stimuli can be endogenous or exogenous. Box 1 presents examples of stressors that can stimulate adrenocortical function. Corticosterone protects the organism against the deleterious effects of stress by balancing the production and action of biologically active substances released during stress episodes, such as catecholamines and prostaglandins [6].

The principal effects of corticosteroids are related to metabolism, immune function, behavior, and electrolyte balance. These effects are summarized in Table 2. Birds differ from mammals in that in some species, corticosterone has both glucocorticoid and mineralocorticoid activity. For example, in free-ranging Mallard ducks living in coastal estuaries and alkaline lake environments, an increase in extracellular sodium or associated anion, or an increase in extracellular osmolality will stimulate the release of ACTH followed by corticosterone. The corticosterone will act as a mineralocorticoid simultaneously on three target organs: small intestine, nasal salt glands, and kidney. In birds that do not have nasal glands and cannot tolerate hyperosmotic drinking water, as in most mammals, corticosterones do not function as mineral-regulating hormones and sodium does not act as a secretogogue for ACTH release [6]. Adrenocortical steroids have both beneficial and

---

Box 1. Stressors in birds [1,5,6,12]

Handling/immobilization
Dietary protein restriction
Food and/or water deprivation
Vitamin A deficiency
Fear
Pain
Depressed liver metabolism of corticosterone
Exercise
Temperature extremes
High-density housing
Noise
Hypovolemia (dehydration, hemorrhage)
Decreased blood concentration of potassium

Table 2
Major effects of corticosteroids [1,2,5,6,11,12]

	Effect	Consequence
Metabolism	Increased hepatic gluconeogenesis	Hyperglycemia and hyperinsulinemia (with secondary lipogenesis and obesity)
	Reduced peripheral glucose uptake	Glucosuria and polyuria/ polydipsia
	Increased hepatic glycogenesis	
	Reduced protein synthesis	Muscle wasting, delayed
	Increased protein mobilization	growth, weight loss
	Increased peripheral lypolysis	Hepatomegaly, increased
	Increased fatty acid mobilization and oxidation	blood levels of cholesterol, triglycerides, high-density lipoproteins
	Lipogenesis (as a result of hyperinsulinemia)	Increased fat deposition, largely in the abdomen
	Increase food consumption	
	Increase gastric transit time	
Immunity	Involution of the thymus, spleen, bursa of Fabricius	Increased susceptibility to viral, mycoplasma and parasitic infections
	Reduction of number of circulating leukocytes (except heterophils) due to redistribution to secondary lymphoid tissue	
	Suppression of cellular cytotoxicity and lymphoproliferation	
	Suppression of interleukin-2 and interferon-γ	
	Decreased T-cell immunity	
	Decreased antibody production	
	Relative increase in circulating heterophils	Increased resistance to bacterial infections
	Enhanced tracheal mucociliary clearance	
Electrolyte balance	Increased sodium resorption and potassium retention in the kidney tubules (corticosterone)	
	Increased potassium excretion in the renal tubules (aldosterone)	
	Increased water uptake across intestinal mucosa	
	Increased sodium absorption and potassium excretion in the distal intestine (aldosterone)	
	Increased potassium excretion in distal intestine	
	Increased sodium excretion through the nasal gland in hyperosmotic water environment	

Table 2 (*continued*)

	Effect	Consequence
Behavior	Influence or disrupt behavior associated with breeding, rearing of young, territoriality	
	Fearfulness	
	Enhancement of oral stereotypic behavior, such as eating, drinking, and pecking	Stress-related feather picking
	Salt appetite in pigeons (aldosterone)	

deleterious effects in the immune system (see Table 2). The lymphocytes themselves can secrete ACTH and therefore boost circulating corticosterone levels following antigenic challenge. Macrophages are activated as they phagocytize an antigen. The activated macrophages secrete interleukin-1, which increases secretion of CRF and ACTH, and activates lymphocytes, with increased production of ACTH. Prolonged stress before antigenic stimulation may blunt this ACTH and interleukin-1 response. Corticosteroids and ACTH act in a negative feedback manner to regulate and control the production of antibodies by inhibiting lymphocyte activities and reducing their responsiveness to stimuli. In chicken strains with autoimmune disease, there is a significantly lower corticosterone response to antigenic stimuli, with consequent reduced negative feedback of corticosterone on ACTH. This may be the cause of the continuous and pronounced immune response characteristic of autoimmune diseases [12].

Clinical considerations

Adrenocortical disorders

Although adrenal lesions have been described on postmortem examinations in a high percentage of birds, a clinical diagnosis of spontaneous adrenal disease has not been reported in birds [2,6]. The ACTH stimulation test and dexamethasone suppression test used in mammals to diagnose adrenal disease can potentially be used in birds for the diagnosis of both hypoadrenocorticism and hyperadrenocorticism [6].

Hyperadrenocorticism (Cushing's syndrome)

Cushing's syndrome is a commonly recognized endocrine disease in humans and dogs. It can occur as a result of excessive levels of corticosteroids with exogenous or endogenous origin. Excessive endogenous secretion can be secondary to stress or to a primary functional tumor of the adrenal gland, a pituitary tumor that hypersecretes ACTH or ectopic ACTH secretion from a nonpituitary tumor. Exogenous corticosteroids can result in excessive levels of circulating corticosteroids and cause hyperadrenocorticism [13].

Pituitary adenomas are the most commonly reported neuroendocrine tumors in birds. They are most prevalent in budgerigars and cockatiels [2,6,14,15]. Pituitary adenomas occur less frequently in other species of birds and have been reported in a Moluccan cockatoo [16], Amazon parrot, lovebird, canary, and chicken [17]. Pituitary carcinoma and adenocarcinoma have also been reported in budgerigars and in a cockatiel [15,17]. These pituitary tumors can be nonfunctional (Amazon parrot [17]) or hypersecrete ACTH and be associated with bilateral adrenal hyperplasia (Moluccan cockatoo [16], budgerigar [6]). Primary neoplastic diseases of the adrenal gland reported in birds include bilateral adrenal adenoma (budgerigar), unilateral adrenal adenoma (budgerigar, leghorn chicken), adrenal adenoma (pheasant, peafowl), and unilateral adrenocortical carcinoma (pigeon, macaw, duck) [4,6,15,18–20]. Carcinomas can become very large and may metastasize [18]. Heterotopic adrenal tissue may occur in the ovary, with both cortical and chromaffin cell tumors being tentatively identified in this site [6].

As for mammals, exogenous corticosteroids can cause hyperadrenocorticism. Chronic stress may result in adrenal hypertrophy from continual ACTH stimulation [6,14]. Chronic exposure of Herring gulls to South Louisiana crude oil causes adrenal hypertrophy and short-term increases in circulating corticosterone, interpreted as an initial response to acute stress [21]. The response of the HPA system to stress in birds can also be affected by heavy metals, as demonstrated in young White storks (*Ciconia ciconia*) exposed to sublethal levels of lead that respond to stress from handling with higher concentration of corticosterone after handling than nonexposed birds [22].

Clinical signs of pituitary neoplasms are usually secondary to space-occupying effects of the tumor and are characterized by unilateral or bilateral exophthalmia, blindness, and other neurological signs, such as depression, ataxia, seizures, and convulsions [15,17]. Polydipsia and polyuria have been described in some cases, likely related to overproduction of ACTH (with secondary adrenal hyperplasia), excess of growth hormone, or hyposecretion of arginine vasotocin hormone. Similarly, changes in cere and plumage color and quality could be explained by alterations in sex hormone and thyroid hormone production. The affected bird's body condition varies from progressive weight loss as seen in cockatiels to obesity, common in affected budgerigars [17].

The clinical signs of hyperadrenocorticism correspond to the described physiological effects of endogenous steroids in the metabolism, electrolyte balance, behavior, and immune system (see Table 2). The excessive levels of corticosteroids can result in many clinical problems, including weight loss, fatty liver disease, feather picking, reproductive abnormalities, and changes in the hemogram [12,23]. Clinical signs suggestive of Cushing's syndrome include polydipsia, polyuria, polyphagia, hepatopathy, weight loss, muscular weakness and atrophy, intra-abdominal fat accumulation, hyperglycemia, and glucosuria [4,13,14,24]. It is not known if feather loss is associated with excessive corticosterone production [4]. Hyperadrenocorticism can cause the following clinicopathologic abnormalities in mammals: "stress leukogram" (characterized by neutrophilia, lymphopenia, and monocytosis), increased liver enzymes, hyperglycemia, hypophosphatemia, elevated cholesterol and triglyceride concentration, and glucosuria [13]. Similar clinical signs and clinicopathologic findings have been described in birds with presumptive hyperadrenocorticism [6]. In a study evaluating the effects of stress in wild birds, wild-caught Herring gulls developed marked leukocytosis, heterophilia, and anemia within 4 days of captivity and persisted during the 28 days of captivity, despite "normal" behavior by day 3 of captivity. Pectoral muscle decreased by 33% over the 28 days of the study [23].

The number and severity of these findings vary remarkably in the affected animals, which may present with only one or all of the abnormalities listed. The clinical signs and clinicopathologic findings presented are not specific for hyperadrenocorticism.

Antemortem diagnosis of hyperadrenocorticism in mammals is based on history and clinical signs, physical exam findings, routine blood test and urinalysis results, imaging (radiographs, ultrasound, CT and/or MRI), and specific endocrine tests, such as ACTH stimulation test, dexamethasone suppression test, and determination of ACTH concentration [13]. Histopathology of the adrenal gland and/or pituitary gland can confirm the diagnosis. Results of the described diagnostic tests should be interpreted in relation to clinical signs because of the possibility of nonfunctional pituitary and adrenal tumors.

Clinical and laboratory confirmed cases of spontaneous hyperadrenocorticism have not been reported in birds [4,14]. Although clinical signs and postmortem findings in these cases suggested a diagnosis of hyperadrenocorticism, an ACTH stimulation test was not performed antemortem and the diagnosis could not be confirmed. Recently, an ACTH-secreting pituitary adenoma with secondary bilateral adrenal gland hyperplasia was reported in a Moluccan cockatoo. This bird presented clinical signs and clinicopathological findings consistent with hyperadrenocorticism but had a "normal" response to the ACTH simulation test based on published results for the species. Diagnosis was confirmed with necropsy, histopathology, and immunohistochemistry [16].

Treatment options for hyperadrenocorticism in mammals include surgical treatment (hypophysectomy followed by radiation therapy; adrenalectomy) or medical treatment (mitotane, trilostane, ketoconazole) [13]. The small size of birds and monetary constraints make surgical resection and radiation therapy for treatment of pituitary tumors unlikely in birds. Although trilostane and ketoconazole block corticosterone-secreting pathways, potentially reducing corticosterone blood levels, to the author's knowledge, there are no reports of medical (or surgical) treatment of hyperadrenocorticism in birds. This is likely related to the difficulty in achieving an antemortem diagnosis.

Hypoadrenocorticism (Addison's disease)

Hypoadrenocorticism is a syndrome that results from inadequate production of glucocorticoids and/or mineralocorticoids by adrenocortical cells. Primary hypoadrenocorticism occurs with bilateral adrenalectomy or when there is damage of more than 90% of the adrenal cortices. Cell atrophy or necrosis can be induced by autoimmune diseases, neoplasia, inflammation, infectious diseases, amyloidosis, trauma, or drugs (mitotane, trilostane). Secondary hyperadrenocorticism is characterized by deficient production and secretion of ACTH, which leads to atrophy of the adrenal cortices and reduced secretion of glucocorticoids. Mineralocorticoid production remains adequate because ACTH has minor effects on the production of mineralocorticoids. Secondary hyperadrenocorticism can be caused by large nonfunctional tumors in the hypothalamus or pituitary or, more commonly, associated with prolonged suppression of ACTH by drug therapy with glucocorticoids or progestogens [25].

Adrenal disease is found in a significant number of birds at necropsy [14]. A previous survey revealed 41 of 150 cases of adrenal pathology in psittacine species [26]. A more recent retrospective study involving mostly psittacines, nonspecific adrenal degeneration was found in about 30% of the cases of adrenal disease (half of the cases in African gray parrots), while adenitis was present in 27% of the cases [18]. Idiopathic adrenal gland degeneration has been reported in Amazon parrots and African gray parrots, being the only lesion found in some birds with acute death. Histologically, adrenal degeneration is characterized by swelling and vacuolation of adrenocortical cells [27,28]. Cell necrosis can also occur [14]. Infectious adenitis can be secondary to septicemia, avian chlamydiosis, systemic viral diseases (such as with polyomavirus and paramyxovirus), avian tuberculosis, bacterial peritonitis, and bacterial or mycotic air sacculitis [14,18,26,28,29]. Adrenal adenitis is seen in cases of psittacine proventricular dilation disease but the lymphoplasmacytic inflammatory infiltrate is present within the chromaffin cells [18,28]. Amyloidosis of the adrenal gland has been reported in birds, with variable loss of both cortical and chromaffin cells [28]. Adrenal pathology is also seen in other groups of birds, including passerines, raptors, and waterfowl [26]. Pesticides and pollutants have been showed to be toxic to avian adrenocortical cells. The high lipid content of adrenocortical cells appears to make these cells more susceptible to chemical contaminants, as most of them are hydrophobic. Chronic ingestion of sublethal doses of crude oil in ducks caused structural damage of the inner zone cells of the adrenal cortex, resulting in long-term decreases in circulating corticosterone concentration (despite hypertrophy in an attempt to compensate for impaired function) [30,31]. Exposure of nestling bald eagles to organochlorides depresses corticosterone levels and response to ACTH stimulation [32].

Adrenal insufficiency should be suspected in birds with hyperkalemia, hyponatremia, a sodium to potassium ratio of less than 27:1, anemia, hypoglycemia, hypercalcemia, low urine specific gravity, dehydration, episodes of weakness, and vague gastrointestinal signs such as anorexia, periodic diarrhea, and generalized abdominal tenderness [4,14,26,29]. Adrenal degeneration has been associated with feather loss in a Sulfur-crested cockatoo [29] and a Blue and gold macaw [33]. As with hyperadrenocorticism, not all clinical signs described have to be present in the same individual. It is important to note that these clinical and clinicopathologic findings are also not specific to hypoadrenocorticism and may be seen with renal, gastrointestinal, or hepatic disease.

Diagnosis in mammals is routinely based on clinical signs, baseline blood and urine test abnormalities, and specific endocrine tests, mainly ACTH stimulation test and endogenous ACTH plasma concentration [25]. Despite the high incidence of adrenal disorders on postmortem examination in birds, there is no clinical report, appropriately documented with antemortem baseline blood and specific hormonal testing, of naturally occurring hypoadrenocorticism in birds [14]. It is likely that adrenal deficiency does exist but either the primary systemic disease or adrenal disease rapidly progresses to death before appropriate diagnostic test for hypoadrenocorticism can be performed.

Treatment of hypoadrenocorticism in mammals consists of intravenous saline and glucocorticoid administration in acute phase of the disease, followed by the use of mineralocorticoid maintenance therapy alone or in combination with glucocorticoids (depending on the mineralocorticoid used) [25]. Although experimental adrenalectomy in birds causes acute death due to hyperkalemia and hyponatremia, affected birds can be maintained with high NaCl intake and corticosterone injections [6]. Protocols for treatment of adrenal insufficiency in psittacine birds have been suggested, using dexamethasone (2 mg/mL) 0.1 to 0.2 mL and fludrocortisone (0.1-mg tablet) 0.25 to 1.00 tablet per 4 oz drinking water [26]. It is important to note that diagnosis of hypoadrenocorticism in this reference was based on failure of cortisol blood levels, not corticosterone to rise after ACTH stimulation test.

ACTH stimulation test in birds

Confirmation of a clinical suspicion of adrenal insufficiency or Cushing's syndrome can be made by determining the plasma *corticosterone* concentration *before* and *after* ACTH stimulation.

Several early case reports of adrenal insufficiency in psittacine birds were based on failure of basal cortisol levels to rise following an ACTH stimulation test [26,29]. In all avian species tested, corticosterone, not cortisol, is the main corticosteroid produced by the "adult" adrenal gland. In ACTH stimulation tests performed in psittacines and raptors, corticosterone concentrations increased significantly after ACTH stimulation while cortisol concentrations remained low [8–10]. For this reason, corticosterone should be the hormone measured if an ACTH stimulation test is performed [2,4,6–10,14,34].

Diagnosis of hyperadrenocorticism in a Scarlet macaw was based on "elevated" levels of corticosterone in a single blood sample without an ACTH stimulation test [20]. As described before, the blood concentration of corticosterone in birds varies significantly with time of the day, season, reproductive activity, genetics, and degree of stress (eg, handling, food deprivation). Also, the concentration of corticosterone in the plasma reflects not only the rate of synthesis and the distribution of hormone within the organism, but also the rate at which it is metabolized and removed from the circulation. In the ducks chronically exposed to crude oil, reduced blood concentrations of corticosterone were presumptively not only due to adrenocortical cell damage but also to their indirect effects on corticosterone metabolism (mainly liver) [30,31]. Adrenal insufficiency may exist even though an animal has normal resting corticosterone concentrations. Hyperadrenocorticism can also occur with normal resting corticosterone concentration. For this reason, a one-time determination of corticosterone concentration in the blood does not reflect accurately adrenocortical function, for which is required direct stimulation of the adrenal gland with exogenous ACTH and determination of corticosterone before and after ACTH stimulation [35]. Hypoadrenocorticism should be suspected when little or no increase in corticosterone blood levels is seen after ACTH administration, while animals with hyperadrenocorticism present an exaggerated increase in corticosterone after ACTH stimulation. Despite this, an ACTH stimulation test does not distinguish pituitary-dependent hyperadrenocorticism (PDH) from functional adrenal tumor (FAT) and primary from secondary hypoadrenocorticism [13,25].

Protocols for an ACTH stimulation test have been developed for psittacines, raptors, pigeons, chickens, and ducks [7–10,34–36]. ACTH stimulation tests have also been performed in cranes [37]. ACTH stimulation tests can be performed with aqueous porcine ACTH gel (Adrenomone; Burns-Biotec, Omaha, NE now Summit Hill Laboratories, Tinton Falls, NJ; also Acthar gel, Questcor Pharmaceuticals Inc, Union City, CA), aqueous porcine ACTH solution (using ACTH fragment 1-39 powder, Sigma Chemical Company, St Louis, MO) or aqueous synthetic ACTH-cosyntropin (Cortrosyn; Organon, West Orange, NJ; now Amphastar Pharmaceuticals, Rancho Cucamonga, CA; Cortrosyn, Organon, The Netherlands). Natural porcine ACTH solution given at 10 IU/kg to ducks did not produce consistent results [35], but was reliable at 50 IU/bird for ACTH stimulation in chickens [36]. Significant stimulation occurs with both ACTH gel and cosyntropin in all other species of birds tested [4]. To perform an ACTH stimulation test, a baseline blood sample is collected, 16 to 50 units of ACTH are administered intramuscularly, and a second blood sample is collected between 1 and 2 hours after ACTH administration. Blood is collected into EDTA or lithium heparin tubes. Quantification of corticosterone requires an assay specific to this hormone, commonly radioimmunoassay (RIA) [4,14]. Cosyntropin adverse reactions are rare and usually limited to local reaction at the injection site, although systemic hypersensitivity reactions can occur [38]. The only reported reactions to ACTH injections in birds was in cranes given cosyntropin intravenously (IV); some birds presented agitation and regurgitation shortly after ACTH administration [37].

Table 3 summarizes ACTH stimulation protocols and corticosterone concentrations before and after ACTH stimulation for a few avian species. Depending on the dose and route of administration, in general, ACTH causes a peak corticosterone response within 30 to 60 minutes after injection with a return to baseline levels within 120 to 240 minutes. In healthy pigeons, a 10- to 100-fold increase over baseline corticosterone concentrations is considered normal for poststimulation samples [34]. For healthy cockatoos, macaws, Amazon parrots, and lorikeets, the mean post-ACTH corticosterone concentrations were 4 to 14 times the mean baseline concentrations [7]. In normal ducks, a 2- to 6-fold increase in corticosterone concentration was noted 1 hour post-ACTH stimulation [35]. In chickens, a 16-fold increase in corticosterone concentration after ACTH stimulation was considered normal [36]. Cranes receiving cosyntropin IV increased their serum corticosterone up to fivefold above baseline concentrations at

Table 3
Summary of ACTH stimulation test protocols and baseline and post-ACTH stimulation corticosterone concentrations

Species	n	Dose	ACTH used	Pre-ACTH CS (ng/mL)	Post-ACTH CS (ng/mL)	R
Cockatoo	20	15 IU	Cortrosyn	26	108	[8]
Cockatoo	5	15 IU	Cortrosyn	14.5 ± 7.2	45.5 ± 12.9	[39]
Cockatoo with PBFD	10	15 IU	Cortrosyn	23.5 ± 12.0	61.0 ± 24.7	[39]
Cockatoo	7	16 IU	Adrenomune	6.7 ± 2.9	29 ± 13.4	[7]
Green-winged macaw	5	16 IU	Adrenomune	3.1 ± 3.07	18.7 ± 5.7	[7]
Blue and Gold macaw	6	16 IU	Adrenomune	1.83 ± 1.6	25.3 ± 5.5	[7]
Amazon	6	16 IU	Adrenomune	2.66 ± 3.16	32.1 ± 10.7	[7]
Conure (*Aratinga* sp.)	3	16 IU	Adrenomune	2.7±3.1	16.5 ± 10.8	[7]
Lorikeet (*Charmosyna* sp.)	2	16 IU	Adrenomune	1.72 ± 1.89	22.5 ± 3.5	[7]
Red-lored amazon	12	125 µg	Cortrosyn	10.6 ± 3.3	48.9 ± 12.6	[9]
Blue-fronted amazon	12	125 µg	Cortrosyn	20.9 ± 9.3	105.8 ± 17.1	[9]
African gray parrots	12	125 µg	Cortrosyn	22.3 ± 8.3	46.7 ± 12.8	[9]
Pigeon	30	50 or 125 µg	Cortrosyn	3.4 ± 0.4	22–150	[34]
Chicken	5	50 IU	ACTH I-39	1.3	25	[36]
Duck	31	25 µg	Cortrosyn	49.7–87.6	132–312	[35]
Bald eagles	10	125 µg	Cortrosyn	66.4 ± 15.1	130.4 ± 27.1	[10]
Andean condor	4	125 µg	Cortrosyn	83 ± 29.1	111.0 ± 23.3	[10]

Abbreviations: CS, corticosterone blood concentration; n, number of animals in the study; R, reference.

60 minutes post injection, with a return to normal baseline concentrations 180 minutes after ACTH administration [37].

As noted in the presented values, pre and post peak corticosterone concentrations vary significantly among avian species. This is likely due to differences of a variety of factors, including handling and restraint procedures, response of the bird to handling and medical procedures, assay methods, ACTH type used, dose and route of administration, and species response to exogenous ACTH [8,35]. In cranes, physical restraint and IV catheter placement caused an increase in serum corticosterone almost comparable to that induced by ACTH stimulation [37]. In an ACTH stimulation test study in eagles and condors, condors had higher resting corticosterone concentrations and less pronounced increase after stimulation, likely a result of differences in behavior and response to handling [17]. Another cause of variation in the magnitude of response to ACTH stimulation could be related to different sensitivity of the adrenal gland to ACTH at different times of the day, with different photoperiods or physiologic states (reproduction, molt) of the experimental groups. In an experimental setting, laying hens had adrenal sensitivity to ACTH almost two times higher in the morning than in the evening [40], while in captive house sparrows, adrenal sensitivity to ACTH was greatest at night [41]. Studies in pigeons revealed no evidence for diurnal variation in responsiveness to ACTH stimulation [42]. The captive house sparrow experimental study also revealed that the daytime adrenal sensitivity to ACTH was greatest in long-day photoperiods, lower in short-day photoperiod and lowest during molt [41].

Another factor to take into consideration is the sensitivity and specificity of ACTH stimulation test in birds, which has not been determined. In dogs, ACTH stimulation test has a sensitivity of 60% to 85% and the specificity of 85% to 90%, with higher sensitivity for diagnosis of pituitary dependent hyperadrenocorticism (PDH) (85%) than diagnosis of functional adrenal tumors (FAT) (60%) [13]. It is also possible that, as for mammals, false-positive and false-negative ACTH stimulation tests occur in birds. A Moluccan cockatoo with suspected hyperadrenocorticism based on clinical signs and routine blood tests abnormalities showed results to ACTH stimulation test that were considered normal based on data available for the species. Postmortem examination confirmed diagnosis of PDH [16].

Therefore, the presented values should be interpreted and used carefully since ACTH stimulation test and corticosterone assays have not been validated in most species of birds.

A dexamethasone suppression test can be used to evaluate the HPA axis and aid diagnosis of hyperadrenocorticism. In normal dogs, the cortisol concentration decreases 2 to 3 hours after administration of dexamethasone and remains low for up to 24 to 48 hours. With hyperadrenocorticism, the HPA axis is abnormally resistant to the suppressive effects of dexamethasone. Extended low-dose dexamethasone suppression test and high-dose dexamethasone suppression test can be used to differentiate PDH from

FAT [13]. The effects of the dexamethasone suppression test in blood corticosterone concentrations have been investigated in pigeons [43] and chickens [36,44], with this information being potentially useful for application of this test to the diagnosis of adrenal disorders in birds.

In mammals, determination of ACTH concentration is a reliable test for differentiating PDH from FAT and primary from secondary hypoadrenocorticism [13,25]. In cases of FAT, the ACTH concentration is suppressed through negative feedback, while with PDH, ACTH is overproduced by the tumor [13]. With hypoadrenocorticism, primary disease is associated with extremely elevated ACTH concentrations because of the lack of negative feedback, whereas secondary disease is associated with low or undetectable ACTH concentrations [25]. The use of ACTH blood concentration in birds for diagnosis of adrenal disease requires further investigation.

Clinical use of corticosteroids

Glucocorticoid agents are among the most commonly used drugs in veterinary medicine. They exert many effects on nearly every tissue in the body and result in desired and undesired actions. These effects vary with the potency and preparation of the glucocorticoid product, dose and route of administration, duration of glucocorticoid exposure, and individual patient factors. Glucocorticoid drugs can be divided into three groups based on duration of HPA axis suppression, with short-acting glucocorticoids suppressing HPA axis for less than 12 hours and long-acting glucocorticoids suppressing for more than 48 hours. The potency of these products is expressed as it relates to cortisol (Table 4) [45].

Corticosteroids can be used for treating hypoadrenocorticism and for treatment of many nonadrenal disorders in mammals. Their therapeutic use is based on the metabolic, anti-inflammatory, and immunosuppressive effects of glucocorticoids (see Table 2). Glucocorticoids are commonly used for many inflammatory diseases (skin, gastrointestinal tract, eye, respiratory tract, nervous system, joints), for conditions where an immunosuppressive effect is required (autoimmune diseases, organ transplant), and for neoplasia (lymphoma, lymphosarcoma, multiple myeloma, leukemia, mast cell tumors) [45,46]. Indications for use of corticosteroids in birds are similar to mammals; dosages and modes of application are derived from those of mammals [11]. Glucocorticoids, such as dexamethasone, betamethasone, prednisolone, and hydrocortisone, are often used as a doping agent in pigeons in Europe. They are thought to enhance racing performance by inhibiting molt, which result in a full wing during competition. These doping glucocorticoids are administered orally, in the drinking water, or as ophthalmic drops [11,47].

When choosing the treatment protocol, it is important to define the goal of corticosteroid treatment: physiologic mineralocorticoid replacement requires a different drug and lower dose than when an anti-inflammatory effect is needed, which in turn requires a lower dose than when

Table 4
Comparison of the action of synthetic corticosteroids [45,46]

	Equivalent pharmacologic dose, mg	Relative glucocorticoid potency	Relative mineralocorticoid potency	Preparations available
Short-acting				
Hydrocortisone	20	1	2	O, I, topical
Cortisone	25	0.8	2	O, I, OD, OI
Intermediate-acting				
Prednisone	5	4	1	O
Prednisolone	5	4	1	O, I, OD, OI, A
Methyl-prednisolone	4	5	0	O, I, OI, C
Triamcinolone	4	5	0	O, I, OI, C, lotion, foam, spray
Long-acting				
Dexamethasone	0.75	30	0	O, I, OI, C, A, lotion, gel
Betamethasone	0.6	30	0	O, I, OI, C, A, lotion, gel
Paramethasone	2	10	0	O, I
Mineralocorticoids				
Fludrocortisone	2	10	250	O, I, OI, otic suspension
Desoxycorticosterone	0	0	20	O, I

Abbreviations: A, aerosol; C, creams; I, injectable; O, oral; OD, ophthalmic drops; OI, ointment.

immunosuppression is the desired effect. Additional factors to consider are related to the patient (species, concurrent disease), the disease process (acute versus chronic, local versus systemic), and available corticosteroid products (solubility, duration of action, route of administration). Ideally, corticosteroids should be used at the lowest dose and shortest-acting preparation possible to achieve the desired effect and minimize systemic effects [45,46].

Many adverse effects of glucocorticoid therapy have been described in mammals and many of them correlate with the physiologic effects of endogenous corticosteroids, which are the same as the signs and symptoms of Cushing's syndrome. They are summarized in Box 2. In birds, glucocorticoids have been reported to affect body condition/fat deposition; immune function; gonad function; plasma thyroid hormone levels; behavior; temperature regulation; liver; and to induce hyperglycemia, glucosuria, hyperlipidemia, polyuria, polydipsia, and polyphagia [6,11,12,43,48]. As in mammals, glucocorticoids appear to increase the risk of secondary infections. Corticosteroid administration in birds causes suppression of both cell-mediated and humeral immunity. One single dose of corticosteroids has been demonstrated to cause lymphopenia and heterophilia in racing pigeons and chickens. The heterophilia likely does not result in increased resistance to infection because overall immune cell function is impaired [6]. Such immunosuppressive effects can result in secondary fungal, bacterial, viral, and

---

Box 2. Adverse effects of glucocorticoid administration in mammals [45,46]

Iatrogenic Cushing's syndrome
Iatrogenic Addison's disease
Gastrointestinal bleeding/perforation
Thyroid atrophy
Hepatomegaly, vacuolar hepatopathy
Growth retardation, weight loss, muscle atrophy, and wasting
Diabetes mellitus, insulin resistance
Pacreatitis
Immunosuppression with secondary infections
Sodium and fluid retention
Abortion, decreased fertility
Polyuria, polydipsia, polyphagia
Alopecia, skin thinning, delayed wound healing
Hyperlipidemia
Osteoporosis
Psychosis, behavior changes

---

parasitic infections. Repeated dexamethasone injections in young turkeys results in a higher incidence of infections caused by opportunistic bacteria, such as *Escherichia coli* and *Staphylococcus aureus* [49]. In pigeons affected with intestinal coccidea, dexamethasone causes a dose-depended increase in excretion of oocysts. Because monocytes are especially susceptible to the effects of steroids, infections causes by agents that elicit a monocytic response, such as *Aspergillus* spp. and *Mycobacteria* spp, are more likely to develop with corticosteroid treatment [6]. Prolonged use of glucocorticoids has been associated with death secondary to respiratory aspergillosis in Amazon parrots [50], budgerigars [51], and pigeons [11]. By interfering with protein metabolism and amino acid availability, glucocorticoids may affect feather development and induce formation of "stress bars" in feathers developing during corticosteroid treatment [6].

Although iatrogenic hyperadrenocorticism is a common complication of corticosteroid treatment, iatrogenic hypoadrenocorticism can also occur. Pharmacological derivates of cortisol exert a similar negative feedback on the HPA axis, with suppression varying with glucocorticoid potency and route of administration [45]. Rapid withdrawal of exogenous glucocorticoids in a patient with suppression of the HPA axis can result in clinical hypoadrenocorticism [45,46]. When administering glucocorticoids for more than 2 weeks, the dosage should be reduced slowly. Full recovery of prolonged suppression may take 2 to 6 months [46]. Research in pigeons has demonstrated that the HPA axis in this species is more sensitive to suppression by glucocorticoids than that of mammals and that dexamethasone causes a more prolonged suppression than cortisol or prednisolone. Prednisolone caused a more pronounced depression in corticosterone blood levels than cortisol and dexamethasone [43]. The administration of dexamethasone 1 mg/kg for 6 weeks to pigeons resulted in suppression of corticosterone secretion for 6 to 7 weeks after cessation of treatment [11]. Also in pigeons, plasma corticosterone concentrations are suppressed by glucocorticoids in a dose-related manner not only with oral administration, but also with topical administration of eye drops and application to the intact skin of preparations with DMSO [47]. Administration of dexamethasone intravenously or intramuscularly to Barred owls (*Strix varia*) and Red-tailed hawks (*Buteo jamaicensis*) caused decrease in plasma corticosterone concentrations for 18 and 24 hours, respectively, despite the short plasma half-life of the drug (30 to 60 minutes) [51].

The result of these case reports and experimental studies regarding the use of glucocorticoids in birds suggests that birds are more sensitive to the secondary effects of exogenous glucocorticoids than mammals [43,47]. Treatment with glucocorticoids in birds should be limited to specific conditions, such as respiratory disease combined with lung edema or anti-inflammatory/immunosuppressive therapy [50]. Precise dosages of different corticosteroids have not been determined in birds [6]. When glucocorticoids are used in birds, dosage should be lower than in mammals, duration of the treatment limited, short-acting corticosteroids should be used, and topical application chosen when possible to minimize secondary effects [6,50]. Even with topical application in ophthalmic and dermatologic conditions, high blood levels of glucocorticoids can occur [4]. Furthermore, prophylactic administration of antibiotics and antifungal agents should be considered if prolonged corticosteroid treatment is necessary [50].

In some mammals, it has been suggested that glucocorticoids should be administered once a day at the time of peak in plasma corticosterone concentration, when the HPA axis is less sensitive to the suppressive effects of exogenous glucocorticoids. These times are early morning for humans and dogs and evening for nocturnal mammals [43]. Based on similar findings on diurnal variation of corticosterone levels in chickens and pigeons, the same recommendations could be made for diurnal birds. The situation might be reversed in nocturnal species. Another alternative for prolonged treatment is alternate-day treatment at double the daily dose [6]. When the desired therapeutic goal is achieved, treatment should be slowly tapered off to prevent development of iatrogenic hypoadrenocorticism [6,47].

Summary

The avian adrenal parenchyma is composed of an intermingling of adrenocortical and chromaffin tissue, without the distinct histologic regions of outer cortex and inner medulla found in the adrenals of mammals. Corticosterone is the main corticosteroid produced by the adult avian adrenal gland. The secretion of corticosteroids is mainly controlled by the HPA system via ACTH. Avian corticosteroids affect different organs and systems, with actions similar to what is described for mammals. Despite the relatively high incidence of pituitary and adrenal pathology on postmortem examinations in birds, there are no reported cases of hyper- or hypoadrenocorticism with antemortem confirmation. Protocols for an ACTH test have been established for different species of birds. Many factors can affect the obtained results and these tests have not been validated in birds. Based on clinical and experimental data regarding the use of exogenous glucocorticoids in birds, they appear to be more sensitive to the secondary effects of these drugs than mammals. The use of glucocorticoids should be restricted to specific cases. Dosages should be lower than in mammals, the drug given for limited period of time, given once a day in the morning for diurnal species or double the dose and given every other day. Also to reduce the risk and severity of secondary effects, short-acting glucocorticoids should be used. The potential for exacerbation of subclinical infections or induction of iatrogenic hyper- or hypoadrenocorticism increases with prolonged therapy.

Acknowledgments

The author thanks Dr. James Morrisey for his mentorship and help in preparation of this article, and Dr. Simon Starkey for providing some of the references sited in this article.

References

[1] Carsia RV, Harvey S. Adrenals. In: Wittow GC, editor. Sturkie's avian physiology. 5th edition. Orlando (FL): Academic Press; 2000. p. 489–537.
[2] Oglesbee BL, Orosz S, Dorrestein GM. The endocrine system. In: Altman RB, Clubb SL, Dorrestein GD, Quesenberry K, editors. Avian medicine and surgery. Philadelphia: Saunders; 1997. p. 475–88.
[3] Holmes WN, Cronshaw J. Adrenal gland: some evidence for the structural and functional zonation of the steroidogenic tissues. J Exp Zool 1984;232:627–31.
[4] Lothrop CD. Diseases of the endocrine system. In: Rosskopf WJ, Woerpel RW, editors. Diseases of caged and aviary birds. Baltimore (MD): Williams and Wilkins; 1996. p. 368–79.
[5] Freeman BM. Adrenal glands. In: Freeman BM, editor. Physiology and biochemistry of the domestic fowl, vol. 4. New York: Academic Press; 1983. p. 191–209.
[6] Lumeij JT. Endocrinology. In: Ritchie BW, Harrison GJ, Harrison LR, editors. Avian medicine: principles and aplication. Lake Worth (FL): Wingers; 1994. p. 582–606.
[7] Lothrop CD, Olsen JH, Loomis MR, et al. Evaluation of adrenal function in psittacine birds using the ACTH stimulation test. J Am Vet Med Assoc 1985;187(11):1113–5.
[8] Walsh MT, Beldegreen RA, Clubb SL, et al. Effect of exogenous ACTH on serum corticosterone and cortisol concentrations in the Moluccan cockatoo (Cacatua moluccensis). Am J Vet Res 1985;46(7):1584–8.
[9] Zenoble RD, Kemppainen RJ, Young DW, et al. Endocrine responses of healthy parrots to ACTH and thyroid stimulating hormone. J Am Vet Med Assoc 1985;187(11):1116–8.
[10] Zenoble RD, Kemppainen RJ, Young DW, et al. Effect of ACTH on plasma corticosterone and cortisol in eagles and condors. J Am Vet Med Assoc 1985;187(11):1119–20.

[11] Westerhof I. Pituitary-adrenocortical function and glucocorticoid administration in pigeons (*Columba livia domestica*). J Avian Med Surg 1998;12(3):167–77.

[12] Hudelson KS, Hudelson PM. Endocrine considerations. In: Harrison GJ, Lightfoot TL, editors. Clinical avian medicine, vol. 2. Palm Beach (FL): Spix Publishing; 2006. p. 541–57.

[13] Reusch CE. Hyperadrenocorticism. In: Ettinger SJ, Feldman EC, editors. Textbook of veterinary internal medicine, vol. 2. 6th edition. St Louis (MO): Elsevier Saunders; 2005. p. 1592–612.

[14] Rae M. Avian endocrine disorders. In: Fudge AM, editor. Laboratory medicine: avian and exotic pets. Philadelphia: WB Saunders; 2000. p. 76–89.

[15] Latimer KS. Oncology. In: Ritchie BW, Harrison GJ, Harrison LR, editors. Avian medicine: principles and aplication. Lake Worth (FL): Wingers; 1994. p. 640–72.

[16] Starkey SR, Morrisey JK, Stewart JE, et al. Pituitary dependent relative hyperadrenocorticism in a Moluccan cockatoo (*Cacatua moluccensis*). J Am Vet Med Assoc, in press.

[17] Romagnano A, Mashima TY, Barnes HJ, et al. Pituitary adenoma in an Amazon parrot. J Avian Med Surg 1995;9:263–70.

[18] Schimdt RE, Reavill DR. Endocrine lesions in psittacine birds. Proceedings AAV Conference. San Antonio (TX): 2006. p. 27–9.

[19] Garner MM. Overview of tumors: a retrospective study of case submissions to a specialty diagnostic service. In: Harrison GJ, Lightfoot TL, editors. Clinical avian medicine, vol. 2. Palm Beach (FL): Spix Publishing; 2006. p. 566–71.

[20] Cornelissen H, Verhofstad A. Hyperadrenocorticism caused by an adrenal carcinoma in a parrot. Vet Q 1998;20(Suppl 1):S111.

[21] Holmes WN. Some common pollutants and their effects on steroid hormone-regulated mechanisms. In: Scanes CG, Ottinger MA, Kenny AD, et al, editors. Aspects of avian endocrinology: practical and theoretical implications. Lubbock (TX): Texas Tech Press; 1982. p. 365–70.

[22] Baos R, Blas J, Bortolotti GR, et al. Adrenocortical response to stress and thyroid hormone status in free-living nestling white storks (*Ciconia ciconia*) exposed to heavy metal and arsenic contamination. Environ Health Perspect 2006;114(10):1497–501.

[23] Hoffman AM, Leighton FA. Hemograms and microscopic lesions of herring gulls during captivity. J Am Vet Med Assoc 1985;187(11):1125–8.

[24] Lennox AM, Doneley B. Working up polyuria and polydipsia in the parrot. Proceedings AAV Conference. New Orleans (LA): 2004. p. 59–65.

[25] Herrtage ME. Hypoadrenocorticism. In: Ettinger SJ, Feldman EC, editors. Textbook of veterinary internal medicine, vol. 2. 6th edition. St. Louis (MO): Elsevier Saunders; 2005. p. 1612–22.

[26] Rosskopf WJ, Woerpel RW, Richkind M, et al. Pathogenesis, diagnosis, and treatment of adrenal insufficiency in psittacine birds. California Veterinarian 1982;5:26–30.

[27] Schmidt RE. Diseases of Amazon parrots. Proceedings AAV Conference. Monterey (CA): 2005. p. 155–70.

[28] Schmidt RE, Reavill DR, Phalen DN. Endocrine system. In: Pathology of pet and aviary birds. Ames (IA): Blackwell Publishing; 2003. p. 121–30.

[29] Rosskopf WJ, Woerpel RW, Howard EB, et al. Chronic endocrine disorder associated with inclusion body hepatitis in a sulfur-crested cockatoo. J Am Vet Med Assoc 1981;179(11): 1273–6.

[30] Fry DM, Lowenstine LJ. Pathology of common murres and cassin's auklets exposed to oil. Arch Environ Contam Toxicol 1985;14:725–37.

[31] Gorsline J, et al. The effects of south Louisiana crude oil on adrenocortical function. In: Scanes CG, Ottinger MA, Kenny AD, editors. Aspects of avian endocrinology: practical and theoretical implications. Lubbock (TX): Texas Tech Press; 1982. p. 359–64.

[32] Bowerman WW, Mehne CJ, Best DA, et al. Adrenal corticotropin hormone and nestling bald eagle corticosterone levels. Bull Environ Contam Toxicol 2002;68:355–60.

[33] Onderka DK, Claffey FP. Adrenal degeneration associated with feather loss in a macaw. Can Vet J 1987;28(4):193–4.

[34] Lumeij JT, Boschma Y, Mol J, et al. Action of ACTH upon plasma corticosterone concentrations in racing pigeons (*Columba livia domestica*). Avian Pathology 1987;16:199–204.

[35] Spelman LH, Fleming WJ, Davis GS, et al. Effect of exogenous adrenocorticotropic hormone administration on plasma corticosterone concentrations in American black ducks (*Anas rubripes*). J Wildl Dis 1995;31(2):136–41.

[36] Dehnhard M, Schreer A, Krone O, et al. Measurement of plasma corticosterone and fecal glucocorticoid metabolites in the chicken (*Gallus domesticus*), the great cormorant (*Phalacrocorax carbo*), and the goshawk (*Accipiter gentilis*). Gen Comp Endocrinol 2003;131(3): 345–52.

[37] Ludders JW, Langenberg JA, Czekala NM, et al. Serum corticosterone reponse to adrenocorticotropic hormone stimulation in Florida Sandhill cranes. J Wildl Dis 1995;34(4): 715–21.

[38] Cortrosym- cosyntropin for injection [package insert]. Rancho Cucamonga, California: Amphaster Pharmaceuticals, USA; 2005.

[39] Jacobsen ER, Clubb SL, Simpson C, et al. Feather and beak dystrophy and necrosis in cockatoos: clinicopathologic evaluations. J Am Vet Med Assoc 1986;189:999–1006.

[40] Beuving G, Vonder GM. Comparison of the adrenal sensitivity to ACTH of laying hens with immobilization and plasma baseline levels of corticosterone. Gen Comp Endocrinol 1986; 62(3):353–8.

[41] Romero ML, Rich EL. Photoperiodically-induced changes in hypothalamic-pituitary-adrenal axis sensitivity in captive house sparrows (*Passer domesticus*). Comp Biochem Physiol A Mol Integr Physiol 2007;147(2):562–8.

[42] Westerhof I, Lumeij JT. No evidence for diurnal variation in the responsiveness of the pituitary-adrenocortical axis of the pigeon (*Columba livia domestica*) to stimulation with adrenocorticotrophin and vasopressin. Avian Dis 1996;40(2):453–6.

[43] Westerhof I, Van den Brom WE, Mol JA, et al. Sensitivity of the hypothalamic-pituitary-adrenal system of pigeons (*Columba livia domestica*) to suppression by dexamethasone, cortisol, and prednisolone. Avian Dis 1994;38:435–45.

[44] Etches RJ. A radioummunoassay for corticosterone and its application to the measurement of stress in poultry. Steroids 1976;28(6):763–73.

[45] Cohn LA. Glucocorticoid therapy. In: Ettinger SJ, Feldman EC, editors. Textbook of veterinary internal medicine, vol. 1. 6th edition. St. Louis (MO): Elsevier Saunders; 2005. p. 503–8.

[46] Feldman EC. Glucocorticoid therapy. In: Canine and feline endocrinology and reproduction. Philadelphia: WB Saunders; 1987. p. 218–28.

[47] Westerhof I, Pellicaan CH. Effects of different application routes of glucocorticoids on the pituitary-adrenocortical axis in pigeons (*Columba livia domestica*). J Avian Med Surg 1995;9(3):175–81.

[48] Kaufman GE, Paul-Murphy JR, Finnegan M. Preliminary evaluation of dexamethasone on serum hepatic enzymes, glucose, and total protein in red-tailed hawks. In: Redig PT, Cooper JE, Remple ND, et al, editors. Raptor biomedicine. Minneapolis (MN): University of Minnesota Press; 1993. p. 184–7.

[49] Huff GR, Huff WE, Balog JM, et al. The effect of a second dexamethasone treatment on turkeys previously challenged in an experimental *Escherichia coli* respiratory model of turkey osteomyelitis complex. Poult Sci 1999;78(8):1116–25.

[50] Verstappen FA, Dorrestein GM. Aspergillosis in Amazon parrots after corticosteroid therapy for smoke-inhalation injury. J Avian Med Surg 2005;19(2):138–41.

[51] Burns RB, Birrenkott GP. Half-life of dexamethasone and its effects on plasma corticosterone in raptors. Proceedings of the Joint Conference of the American Association of Zoo Veterinarians and the American Association of Wildlife Veterinarians, Toronto, Ontario, Canada: 1988. p. 12–3.

ELSEVIER
SAUNDERS

Vet Clin Exot Anim 11 (2008) 59–82

VETERINARY
CLINICS
Exotic Animal Practice

Calcium Metabolism in Birds

Ricardo de Matos, LMV, DABVP–Avian

Section of Wildlife and Exotic Medicine, Department of Clinical Sciences,
College of Veterinary Medicine, Cornell University, Ithaca, NY 14853-6401, USA

Calcium is the most prevalent mineral in the body and is required in the diet in a greater amount than any other mineral. Calcium provides structural strength and support (bones and eggshell) and plays vital roles in many of the biochemical reactions in the body. The control of calcium metabolism in birds is highly efficient and closely regulated, essential for the high demands of calcium associated with the eggshell calcification and rapid growth rate of young birds. The classic calcium-regulating hormones, parathyroid hormone, calcitonin, and 1,25-dihydroxyvitamin D_3 (calcitriol), are all recognized in birds, although their actions and/or sensitivities can differ from mammals. Estrogen, androgens, and prostaglandins also appear to have an important role in avian calcium metabolism, while calcitonin plays a minor and uncertain role [1]. Calcium dynamics and regulation in birds will be reviewed. Because of the economic status of the poultry industry, most of our present knowledge in calcium homeostasis and requirements refers to galliformes, with only a few recent studies involving companion birds.

Clinical disease associated with calcium disorders in birds will be discussed, including pathophysiology, clinical signs, and diagnosis and treatment of pathologic calcium deficiency and toxicity.

Calcium physiology in birds

Calcium

Calcium exists in three forms in the body: (1) hydroxyapatite (Ca_{10} $(PO_4)_6(OH)_2$) of the bone, (2) intracellular, and (3) extracellular. The bone calcium constitutes about 99% of the total body calcium. Most of the remaining calcium is intracellular, with less than 0.1% of the calcium in the

---

E-mail address: rd95@cornell.edu

1094-9194/08/$ - see front matter © 2008 Elsevier Inc. All rights reserved.
doi:10.1016/j.cvex.2007.09.005   *vetexotic.theclinics.com*

body in the extracellular fluid. The extracellular calcium is found in three different forms: (1) ionized calcium, (2) calcium bound to proteins, and (3) calcium bound to anions [2].

The ionized calcium is the physiologically active form, with important roles in bone homeostasis, muscle and nerve conduction, blood coagulation, eggshell calcification, and control of hormone secretions such as vitamin D_3 and parathyroid hormone (PTH). Mammals have about 50% of the extracellular calcium in this form [2], whereas in birds, the ionized form ranges from 20% to 60% of the extracellular calcium [3]. Despite this, the absolute values of ionized calcium in birds are comparable to mammals. The ionized calcium concentration appears to be maintained within a tight range in the normal individual. Any major change in the serum-ionized calcium is likely to be clinically significant. Only this fraction of the extracellular calcium is regulated by the interaction of PTH, calcitonin, and vitamin D_3 metabolites in response to changing demands [4].

Approximately 40% of the extracellular calcium is protein bound, mainly to albumin and vitellogenin in birds, and considered to be physiologically inactive (unable to diffuse across capillary membranes). Protein-bound calcium serves as a storage pool or buffering system for ionized calcium. Any change in the serum albumin levels will directly affect the total calcium levels [2,4,5].

The remaining extracellular calcium is bound to interstitial ions (lactate, citrate, bicarbonate), able to diffuse across capillary membranes as ionized calcium. The significance of this calcium fraction is currently unknown [2].

Calcium homeostasis in birds is closely regulated by PTH, calcitonin, vitamin D_3, and sex hormones, acting on the main target organs of liver, kidney, gastrointestinal tract, and bone. Avian calcium metabolism is characterized by several unique characteristics related mainly to the ability of this class to lay large megalecithal eggs with calcified eggshell [1]. The amount of calcium in each egg typically represents about 10% of the total body calcium stores of a chicken. This value increases to 20% in Zebra finches, since smaller birds lay proportionally larger eggs with more shell [1,3]. The calcium required for eggshell calcification is mainly obtained by increased intestinal absorption (up to 70% when compared with 10% to 20% in humans) and resorption of the highly labile reservoir found in the medullary bone, which develops in egg-laying female birds in response to the activity of gonadal steroids [3]. The domestic chicken can respond to hypocalcemic challenges within minutes, while similar challenges in mammals can take over 24 hours [6].

Parathyroid hormone and parathyroid gland

The parathyroid tissue consists of 1 to 2 pairs of glands located caudal to the thyroid glands on either side of the thoracic inlet. Each gland consists of only *chief cells*, with the oxyphil cells of mammalian parathyroids being absent. The chief cells produce PTH in response to hypocalcemia [1,7].

Avian PTH has a different structure than mammalian PTH (88 amino acid chain versus 84 in mammals) but with great similarity in the most biologically active region of the hormone (1 to 34 segment) [1]. This characteristic has been useful for determination of blood concentration of avian PTH using mammalian assays [4]. The concentration of PTH in birds is believed to be low when compared with mammals, with elevation during egg-shell calcification [1].

The major physiological stimulus for PTH secretion is a fall in plasma calcium concentration, while a rise in calcium suppresses it [1]. PTH exerts direct effects on bone and kidney and indirect effects on the intestine through vitamin D_3. PTH elevates plasma calcium by (1) increasing tubular reabsorption of calcium, thus decreasing calcium loss in the urine (and increasing urinary loss of PO_4); (2) increasing bone resorption; and (3) accelerating the formation of $1,25\text{-}(OH)_2\text{-}D_3$ by the kidney [2].

PTH promotes calcium absorption from the bone by affecting cell spread area in avian osteoclasts and inducing rapid changes in calcium transfer by osteoblasts and osteocytes. Birds appear to be more sensitive to PTH than mammals, responding to intravenous injections of the hormone with a rise in blood calcium in minutes, when compared with hours or days in mammals. It is still unknown why birds respond so quickly to PTH. One proposed hypothesis is that PTH signals bone-lining cells (osteoclasts and osteoblasts) to alter their size and shape and migrate to and from areas of the bone surface where high- or low-affinity binding sites for calcium are located. The hypercalcemic effects of PTH are greater in egg-laying hens than in males because of either an increase in calcium-binding proteins in the plasma or presence of additional PTH receptors in the medullary bone and oviduct [1]. A study in ostriches revealed a positive and significant correlation between high levels of PTH in laying ostriches and increased hatchability and production [8]. The importance of PTH in calcium metabolism in birds is proven by the occurrence of fatal hypocalcemia in birds subject to parathyroidectomy [9].

Parathyroid hormone–related peptide (PTHrP) is another member of the PTH family. It was originally discovered as a cause of malignancy-associated hypercalcemia in humans. The hormone has a distinct structural homology with PTH and they share a common receptor. As with PTH, there is homology in the 1 to 34 segment between mammalian and avian PTHrP. In mammals, PTHrP is produced widely in the body and has numerous actions in the fetus and adult organism, many in common with PTH (regulation of calcium metabolism). PTHrP is expressed in many tissues in chick embryos, with effects on bone resorption. Concentrations of PTHrP in the egg-laying hen transiently increase as the egg moves through the oviduct, gradually returning to normal during the calcification period. In the oviduct, this hormone has a potential role of local modulator of vascular smooth muscle tension and shell gland motility during egg laying [1]. Malignancy-associated hypercalcemia has not been reported in birds [5].

Calcitonin and ultimobranchial glands

The ultimobranchial glands are anatomically distinct asymmetrical paired glands positioned caudal to the parathyroid glands in the thoracic inlet. Histologically, these glands are made up of two distinct cell types: the principal cells, very similar to the mammalian thyroid C-cells (possessing small intracytoplasmic granules), and a second morphologically distinct endocrine cell type, with larger intracytoplasmic granules [1]. Despite the differences, both cells appear to be responsible for the production of calcitonin (CT) [10]. In pigeons and turtle doves, CT is also produced by islets of cells within the thyroid gland [11]. The chicken calcitonin 32–amino acid sequence is different from other species, giving rise to differences in bioactivity [1,10].

CT secretion is regulated primarily by rising plasma calcium levels. In mammals the hypocalcemic (and hypophosphatemic) action of CT is based on inhibition of osteoclastic bone resorption [1,12]. Most mammalian osteoclasts examined have CT receptors [12]. At high doses, calcitonin may also promote urinary calcium excretion.

The precise role of calcitonin in avian calcium homeostasis is still controversial. Calcitonin circulates at much higher levels in birds than in mammals [1]. CT binding sites have been demonstrated in the kidneys and bone of chickens and quails [1,13]. In contrast to mammals, administration of calcitonin to eucalcemic birds does not create hypocalcemia. Plasma calcitonin levels do increase significantly in male Japanese quail following injections of calcium [1]. Research in egg-laying chickens and Japanese quail have found higher blood concentrations of CT when shell calcification was not taking place (immediately before or after oviposition), presumably because calcium is still being absorbed from the intestines and mobilized from the bone at a high rate without being removed from the blood by the shell gland [6]. These findings in the experimental models support the theory that calcitonin's function in birds lies specifically in the control of hypercalcemia and in the protection of the bone against excessive calcium resorption. Despite the presence of CT receptors in the kidneys, the role of CT in regulating renal production of vitamin D_3 is still controversial [1,14]. In egg-laying chickens, the binding affinity and capacity of the CT receptors appears to be modulated by sex hormones [13].

Total excision of the ultimobranchial gland in chickens does not affect plasma calcium levels, bone metabolism, egg production, or calcification. Calcitonin levels were not measured during this study, so accessory C-cells could be producing adequate levels of CT in ultimobranchialectomy birds, resulting in no differences of the parameters monitored between these birds and the controls [6].

Calcitonin gene–related peptide (CTGRP) is a neuropeptide derived from the same gene as CT but found only within the central and peripheral nervous system. CTGRP is a potent vasodilator and is implicated in neurotransmission and modulation. Chick, rat, and mouse bones contain cells in osteoblast-rich populations that respond specifically to CTGRP by inhibiting bone resorption [1].

Vitamin D_3

Vitamin D is a steroid hormone that has several forms. The two most important forms of vitamin D are vitamin D_3 and vitamin D_2. Unlike mammals, where the two forms of vitamin D are equivalent in biological activity, many bird species discriminate between vitamin D_3 and D_2. Vitamin D_2, which occurs naturally in plants as ergocalciferol, has only one tenth the efficacy of vitamin D_3 in these species [15]. This is believed to be because of a lower affinity to plasma vitamin D binding proteins with consequent rapid conjugation and excretion in the bile [6,16]. This lower affinity has been demonstrated in 18 species (including 1 psittacine) in 11 orders of birds, and it is assumed to occur in all bird species [16].

Vitamin D_3 plays an important role in calcium homeostasis through its actions on the kidney, intestine, oviduct, and bone. More recent studies found vitamin D_3 also influences the immune system and skin and cancer cells [16–18].

Unlike other fat-soluble vitamins, vitamin D is not primarily stored in the liver but distributed relatively evenly among the lipid components of various tissues [16].

The vitamin D_3 metabolism of birds has been extensively reviewed [1,12,15,16]. Fig. 1 summarizes vitamin D_3 metabolism. Provitamin D (7-dehydrocholesterol) is formed from cholesterol in the liver and secreted onto the skin and, to a less degree, the uropygeal gland [1,16,19]. Conversion of the provitamin D to cholecalciferol (vitamin D_3) occurs by the action of UV-B light, especially in the featherless areas of the skin. Birds do not ingest nutritionally significant amounts of cholecalciferol during the preening process. Cholecalciferol can also be obtained in the diet, usually from marine fish products. Vitamin D_3 supplied in the diet can be absorbed with 60% to 70% efficiency in birds [16]. Cholecalciferol (vitamin D_3) is subsequently activated by a two-stage hydroxylation process. The initial hydroxylation at the 25 position occurs in the liver to form 25-(OH)-D_3 (calcidiol). This reaction is rapid and neither tightly regulated nor influenced by calcium or phosphorus plasma levels, with most cholecalciferol being converted to 25-OH-D_3 [2,16]. It has been demonstrated in chickens that 25-hydroxylation of vitamin D_3 can also occur to a lesser degree in the kidney and intestine [6]. The 25-OH-D_3 is the major circulating form of vitamin D_3 and serves as a pool for further activation or catabolism [2].

The 25-OH-D_3 is transported to the kidney via carrier proteins and converted either to 1,25-(OH)$_2$-D_3 (calcitriol) or 24,25-(OH)$_2$-D_3, the two active metabolites of cholecalciferol in the domestic fowl [15]. The 1,25-(OH)$_2$-D_3 is the most metabolically active form of vitamin D, being 500 to 1000 times

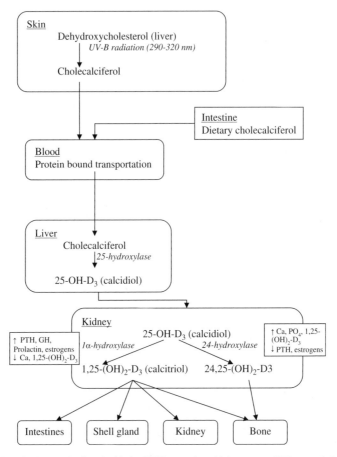

Fig. 1. Vitamin D metabolism in birds. PTH, parathyroid hormone; GH, growth hormone; PO₄, phosphate; Ca, calcium; ↓, up-regulation; ↑, down-regulation.

more active than the other metabolites [2,16]. The hydroxylation at position 1 is a slow and well-regulated process, with PTH, calcium, phosphorus, 1,25-$(OH)_2$-D_3 itself, estrogens, prolactin, and growth hormone being involved. Hypocalcemia, which causes an increase in PTH, will result in up-regulation of hydroxylation at position 1. When the concentration of calcium is normal or high, hydroxylation at position 24 is up-regulated while 1-alpha hydroxylase activity is decreased. In these situations, the major hydroxylation product of 25-OH-D_3 is 24,25-$(OH)_2$-D_3 [2,6]. Thus, under normal physiological circumstances, both dihydroxylated metabolites are being produced.

Vitamin D_3 and its metabolites are transported in the blood by plasma albumins in most birds and also by alpha and beta globulins in a few avian species. The affinity of these proteins to 25- and 24,25-$(OH)_2$-D_3 is similar and about 10 times higher than for 1,25-$(OH)_2$-D_3. The concentration of vitamin D_3-carrying albumins is much higher in egg-laying birds [1,6].

A unique vitamin D–binding protein is synthesized in laying females, with higher affinity for vitamin D_3 than for 25-OH-D_3, delivering vitamin D_3 to the follicle for deposition into the egg yolk [16].

The main target organs for vitamin D_3 are the intestine, bone, and kidney. Most 1,25-$(OH)_2$-D_3 effects in calcium homeostasis are attributed to calcium absorption [12].

The 1,25-$(OH)_2$-D_3 facilitates the absorption of dietary calcium across the duodenum and jejunum wall by increasing synthesis of calcium-binding proteins, mainly calbindin-D_{28k} [1,16,20]. A similar or identical calbindin protein is also present in the distal portion of the uterus (oviduct) of domestic fowl, with levels rising during egg laying; this protein appears to be necessary for translocation of calcium across the oviductal wall. Although the uterus of the laying hen contains receptors for 1,25-$(OH)_2$-D_3, it is believed that oviductal calbindin production is controlled mostly by sex hormones and not by 1,25-$(OH)_2$-D_3, as the production of the intestinal calbindin [1,20]. Calbindin-D_{28k} protein is also found in the kidney, bone, parathyroid gland, pancreas, and chorioallantoic membrane [15].

The effects of 1,25-$(OH)_2$-D_3 in the bone are dependent on blood calcium and phosphorus levels. In eucalcemic patients, this metabolite stimulates bone formation by inducing synthesis of multiple bone proteins produced by osteoblasts [2]. In periods of hypocalcemia (increased levels of PTH) and hypophosphatemia (increased levels of growth hormone), 1,25-$(OH)_2$-D_3 has an opposite effect, promoting osteoclast differentiation and activation with release of calcium and phosphorus into circulation [2,16].

The effects of 1,25-$(OH)_2$-D_3 in the kidney are also dependent on the levels of circulating PTH. With hypocalcemia and in the presence of PTH, this metabolite decreases renal excretion of calcium by increasing tubular resorption. In the absence of PTH, calcium excretion is not affected. The metabolite 1,25-$(OH)_2$-D_3 also inhibits the 25-OH-D_3-1α-hydroxylase in the renal tubule, preventing its own overproduction. Calcitriol (1,25-$(OH)_2$-D_3) also down-regulates the production of PTH in the parathyroid gland, directly and indirectly, by increasing serum calcium concentration [2].

Additional organs with receptors for vitamin D in birds include pancreas, pituitary, and chorioallantoic membrane [15].

Avian keratinocytes and activated macrophages also have the capacity to convert 25-OH-D_3 to 1,25-$(OH)_2$-D_3, a conversion that it is not under the same regulatory factors that modulate the renal 25-OH-D_3-1-hydroxylase. The macrophage-produced 1,25-$(OH)_2$-D_3 appears to have an anti-inflammatory activity and mediates the differentiation of monocytes into osteoclasts [16,21].

The 24,25-$(OH)_2$-D_3 metabolite, although considered the first stage of vitamin D inactivation, inhibits the secretion of PTH (in mammals), is essential for normal growth plate chondrocyte development, and appears to be important in the egg-laying fowl [12,15]. Its direct effect in the bone remains controversial [2,6].

Sex hormones

Estrogen affects calcium metabolism at multiple levels, most of them related to increased calcium storage, mobilization, and transportation (Table 1).

As described above, the amount of calcium in a single chicken egg corresponds to approximately 10% of the total body reserve of calcium. The two main sources of calcium for eggshell formation are bone and dietary calcium [20]. The relative importance of the two organs as a source of calcium depends on the availability of dietary calcium. For example, the medullary bone contributes 30% to 40% of the calcium necessary for a single egg when the concentration of calcium in the food is 2%. The bone contribution can be higher when birds are fed diets with a lower concentration of calcium or during the night, when generally no calcium is consumed and most of the shell calcification occurs in chickens [3,6,20]. Despite this, the total amount of medullar bone is sufficient to supply calcium for about one eggshell. Dietary calcium is then essential to complement and restore the medullary bone reserve before and after shell calcification occurs [3]. Studies have shown that, when given the opportunity, laying hens will preferentially consume diets with higher calcium concentration, especially in the evening [3,6].

At the onset of sexual maturity, with the rise of estrogen concentration in circulation, the function of osteoblasts changes from forming lamellar cortical bone to producing spicules of nonstructural medullary bone in the endosteal surface than can fill the entire bone cavity [22]. Medullary bone formation may be initiated by the sex hormones without the presence of vitamin D_3 but complete mineralization can only occur if vitamin D_3 levels are adequate [23]. Medullary bone is radiographically most prominent in the pelvic limb long bones (femur and tibiotarsus) but can also occur in the thoracic limb long bones (humerus, radius, and ulna) and in other areas of the skeleton [3,22,24]. Medullary bone formation starts around 2 weeks before initiation of egg laying and can be responsible for a 25% increase in the dry fat-free skeletal weight [6].

Table 1
Summary of the effects of estrogen in calcium metabolism [10,13]

Target organ	Effect
Liver	Increased formation of calcium-binding proteins (albumin, vitellogen)
	Stimulation of 25-hydroxylation of vitamin D_3
Kidney	Activation of 25-OH-D_3-1α-hydroxylase (with prolactin)
	Down-regulation of 25-OH-D_3-24R-hydroxylase
	Up-regulation of PTH receptors
Intestines	Up-regulation of mucosal 1,25-$(OH)_2$-D_3 receptors increasing calcium absorption
	Synthesis of calbindin-D_{28k} with 1,25-$(OH)_2$-D_3
Bone	Formation and mobilization of medullary bone
Other effects	Protects vitamin D_3 and 25-OH-D_3 from degradation

The formation of medullary bone, also known as medullary hyperostosis or osteomyelosclerosis, is unique to birds and crocodilians and constitutes a labile source of calcium for eggshell formation at periods when dietary supply is insufficient [3,22]. During the ovulation-oviposition cycles, periods of intense medullary bone formation alternate with periods of severe bone depletion, although some degree of medullary bone formation takes place continuously. In hens fed a high-calcium diet, the medullary bone is replenished with calcium, while hens on a low-calcium diet will experience erosion of the cortical bone while medullary bone is maintained in a fairly constant amount [6,20]. PTH and 1,25-$(OH)_2$-D_3 are responsible for calcium mobilization from medullary bone [6].

When the hen goes out of lay and estrogen levels decline, the osteoblast activity is reversed to forming lamellar cortical bone. Medullary bone gradually disappears and structural bone formation recommences [3].

Under conditions of low calcium in the diet, the regulatory effects of estrogens in calcium metabolism are reduced or absent [25].

Androgens also participate in the development of medullary bone, but do not have a major role in calcium homeostasis [26]. Prostaglandins can also facilitate bone resorption, with hypercalcemic effects in the bone similar to PTH and vitamin D_3 metabolites [1,6]. Prostaglandins may also play a role in calcium secretion in the shell gland [6].

Calcium metabolism of the embryo

Calcium homeostasis of the embryo is regulated tightly by the vitamin D endocrine system, which becomes competent in the chicken embryo at 6 to 8 days of incubation. Vitamin D_3 is present in the yolk of the egg and is absorbed by the embryo, with activating hydroxylation occurring in the mesonephric kidney. 1,25-$(OH)_2$-D_3 mediates the uptake of yolk calcium by the yolk sac membrane in the initial stages of development. As incubation progresses, the developing embryo requires larger amounts of calcium for skeletal development. At this time, 1,25-$(OH)_2$-D_3 promotes the absorption of calcium from the shell via the chorioallantoic membrane. Altricial species begin mobilizing calcium from the shell later during development and at a slower rate than precocial species, resulting in chicks with less mineralized bones at hatching. Toward the end of embryo development, calcium in excess mobilized from the shell is transferred back into the yolk for use following hatching [3,16].

As mentioned above, PTH, vitamin D_3, CT, and sex hormones interact to achieve calcium homeostasis. In summary:[1,2,6]

> In eucalcemic states, vitamin D plays an important role in the intestinal absorption of calcium and phosphorus, which are essential for bone and eggshell mineralization. In egg-laying birds, estrogen and androgens are responsible for the formation of medullary bone, a labile reservoir of calcium for the very high demand period of eggshell calcification.

In hypocalcemic states, PTH and $1,25\text{-}(OH)_2\text{-}D_3$ restore blood calcium by increasing calcium absorption from the intestine, increasing bone resorption and decreasing calcium excretion in the kidneys (Fig. 2). Estrogen in egg-laying birds complements the activity of these two hormones, allowing fast mobilization of calcium in periods of high demand (eggshell calcification). The domestic chicken can respond to hypocalcemic challenges within minutes, while similar challenges in mammals can take over 24 hours.

In hypercalcemia states, there is decreased synthesis of PTH and $1,25\text{-}(OH)_2\text{-}D_3$, with $25\text{-}OH\text{-}D_3$ being hydroxylated mainly to $24,25\text{-}(OH)_2\text{-}D_3$. Calcitonin is released to minimize the magnitude of hypercalcemia possibly by decreasing bone resorption. The plasma calcium concentration is restored by increasing urinary excretion, decreasing intestinal absorption, and a higher ratio of bone formation:bone resorption (Fig. 3).

Dietary requirements

Calcium

Most of the information available on dietary requirements of calcium, vitamin D_3, and phosphorus is based on work with poultry. Calcium dietary requirements vary with species, age, breeding status, and dietary levels of vitamin D. Egg-laying birds and growing birds require more calcium than adult nonbreeding birds. The recommended levels for growing chicks is 1% and for turkey poults is 1.2%, with values dropping for both species

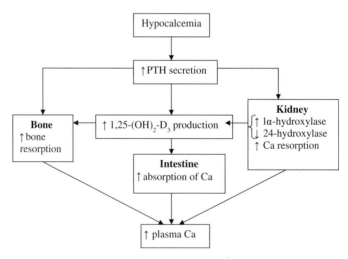

Fig. 2. The control of hypocalcemia. Calcium blood concentrations are restored mainly by the actions of PTH (parathyroid hormone) and $1,25\text{-}(OH)_2\text{-}D_3$ in the bone, kidneys, and intestinal tract.

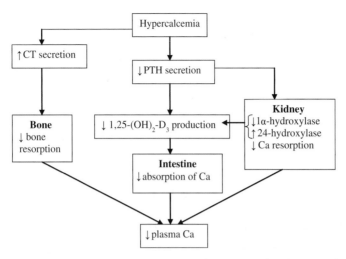

Fig. 3. The control of hypercalcemia. The plasma calcium is restored by increasing the urinary excretion, decreasing intestinal absorption and by reducing bone resorption (with normal rate of bone mineralization). PTH, parathyroid hormone; CT, calcitonin.

after 4 weeks of age. Presumably, fledglings of altricial species have higher dietary calcium requirements when compared with precocial species because of the lower calcification of the skeleton at hatch and faster growth rate. Smaller birds lay proportionally larger eggs than larger birds, and small eggs have proportionally more shell. Laying chickens should be offered a diet containing about 2% calcium, up to 3.25% in prolific egg-laying hens, while laying turkeys require 2.55% [16,24,27]. The calcium requirement for egg-laying cockatiels is 0.35% and for budgies is 0.85% [27]. Within similar size birds, altricial bird species produce relatively smaller eggs, requiring lower calcium concentrations in their diet during egg laying [16]. Suggested general optimum calcium levels for maintenance are between 0.3% and 0.7% [28], with levels above 0.7% being associated with higher risk of toxic effects in some species [29,30]. Most formulated feeds provide calcium percentages higher than 0.7%. The recommended calcium:phosphorus (Ca:P) ratio for birds ranges from 1:1 to 2:1 [31].

Vitamin D

Vitamin D_3 (cholecalciferol) can be obtained from the diet or from exposure to direct UV-B light. Birds with adequate exposure to direct sunlight do not have a requirement for vitamin D. In chickens, 11 to 30 minutes of exposure to direct sunlight is sufficient for endogenous production of vitamin D [16]. Because of differences in natural habitat, South American parrot species, such as macaws and Amazons, do not appear to be as dependent on UV-B light for maintaining adequate levels of vitamin D as African gray parrots [4]. A recent study with captive African gray parrots has shown that supplementary artificial UV-B lighting significantly increases the serum ionized calcium and 25-OH-D_3 concentrations, independent of the calcium or vitamin D_3 content of the diet being fed [32].

For birds kept indoors, vitamin D_3 has to be supplied in the diet. Vitamin D_2 is considered an ineffective nutritional supplement for all avian species because of its lower affinity for vitamin D binding proteins and faster excretion when compared with vitamin D_3. Phytoplankton and zooplankton are rich in vitamin D_3 and, consequently, marine fish are an excellent source of vitamin D_3. Other vertebrate prey may have marginally low vitamin D_3 levels considering the requirements of birds not exposed to sunlight. Vitamin D_3 (cholecalciferol) is typically used to supplement avian diets. Some poultry feeds are supplemented with 25-OH-D_3. Supplementation with 1,25-$(OH)_2$-D_3 is not commonly done because it does not support normal embryonic development and can result in high probability of toxicity [16]. Vitamin D_3 can be absorbed from the intestine with 60% to 70% efficacy in birds [4].

Dietary vitamin D requirements vary with species, age, breeding status, production objective (egg production, maximum growth, fertility, hatchability, and so forth), and with calcium and phosphorus levels in the diet. The vitamin D requirement is increased when the dietary level of calcium is low or when the Ca:P ratio is low or high [16]. The dietary requirement for vitamin D in chickens ranges from 300 IU/kg of feed for egg type white breeders to 1200 to 2800 IU/kg of feed for broiler breeders [33]. Recommended levels of vitamin D_3 for the turkey are 900 IU/kg of feed and for the Japanese quail are 1200 IU/kg of feed [4]. As mentioned above, because of differences in natural habitat, Amazon and macaw species may have a reduced requirement for vitamin D when compared with African gray parrots or may metabolize it in a different manner because of their relatively reduced UV light exposure. This could also explain the higher susceptibility of macaws to vitamin D toxicity [32]. Optimum and toxic levels of vitamin D_3 in the diet for companion birds have not been established and care should be taken when extrapolating vitamin D_3 requirements information from poultry to other species of birds [34,35]. Some formulated diets, including psittacine diets, exceed these recommended levels for poultry, with a potential increase in the risk of toxicity [28].

Clinical considerations

Diagnosis of calcium metabolism disorders

Diagnosis of calcium disorders is routinely based on history, clinical signs, physical examination, blood tests, and radiographic findings. Determination of ionized calcium and blood levels of PTH and vitamin D_3 can potentially aid the diagnosis of calcium metabolism disorders.

Calcium

Most laboratories provide clinicians with values of total blood calcium, which includes ionized, protein-bound, and complexed calcium. The measurement of blood concentration of calcium must be evaluated carefully since (1) it is common to find normal total calcium concentrations within reference range for the species even when history, physical exam findings, and imaging suggest calcium disorders and (2) hyper- or hypocalcemia can be caused by many conditions not directly related with calcium disorders (Table 2). For example, egg-laying birds frequently have elevated total blood calcium concentration associated with increased concentration of carrier proteins (and of the protein-bound calcium fraction), calcium mobilization from medullary bone and lipemic interference [4,36]. In small animal clinical pathology, the calcium concentration can be adjusted to the total protein or albumin concentrations when these values are abnormal using standard formulas [2]. Recent research in dogs has shown that these adjustment formulas are not very accurate and also that total calcium or adjusted calcium levels cannot be used to predict ionized calcium concentrations accurately [37]. The relationship between plasma total calcium concentration and total protein and albumin concentrations has been investigated in several bird species. No positive correlation was found between albumin or total protein concentration and calcium concentration in Amazon parrots [38]. African gray parrots presented conflicting results in 2 separate studies [38,39]. In ostriches and captive peregrine falcons, a significant correlation was found between total calcium and total protein concentrations, with correction formulas for each species being proposed [40,41]. One author states that because analyzed derived albumin levels are artifactually low in birds, it is useless to use these formulas based on inaccurate albumin concentration [36]. Even if corrected, total plasma calcium levels do not provide information regarding ionized calcium concentration, the physiologically active and hormone-regulated fraction of extracellular calcium [42,43].

For these reasons, the determination of serum-ionized calcium provides a more precise estimate of an individual's calcium status, especially in cases of abnormal protein concentration and metabolite or electrolyte imbalances [15]. Ionized calcium levels are not affected by increased or decreased

Table 2
Causes of hypocalcemia and hypercalcemia in birds [4,5,42]

	Hypocalcemia	Hypercalcemia
Primary	Nutritional	Nutritional
	Excess dietary phosphorus	Excess dietary calcium
	Calcium deficiency	Excess dietary vitamin D_3
	Hypovitaminosis D	
	Chronic egg laying	
Secondary	Hypoalbuminemia	Hyperalbuminemia
	Use EDTA collection tubes	Hemolysis
	Hemolysis	Bacterial contamination
	Bacterial contamination	Lipemia
	Sample dilution	

concentration of calcium-binding proteins [4]. In poultry, ionized calcium levels during egg laying are similar to the non–egg-laying period, unlike total calcium levels, although they vary through the ovulatory cycle [20,44]. A recent study in healthy African gray parrots indicated a narrow variation in ionized calcium concentration but a wide variation in total calcium levels due to variation in protein concentration between birds [39].

Limitations to the use of ionized calcium for diagnosis of calcium disorders are the need of special equipment and the effect of blood pH in the ionized calcium levels, potentially requiring immediate analysis. The binding reaction between calcium and albumin is strongly pH dependent, with a decrease in sample pH resulting in an ionized hypercalcemia due to decreased protein binding. Blood samples for ionized calcium determination should be collected into heparin, refrigerated immediately, and analyzed as soon as possible. Silicone separator tubes should not be used because the release of calcium from the silicone gel will cause an increase in ionized calcium concentration. Refrigeration will limit glycolysis by the red blood cells, which can decrease the sample's pH because of lactic acid production. Prolonged contact with CO_2 in the air will also cause a reduction in the pH of the sample. Since ionized calcium and pH are more stable in serum than in whole or heparinized blood, serum should be used if a prolonged storage period before analysis is expected [2]. A recent study in dogs evaluated the effects of storage temperature and time between collection and analysis of ionized calcium. It concluded that if the sample is obtained, handled, and stored anaerobically, ionized calcium concentration can be accurately determined after 72 hours at 23°C or 4°C or after 7 days at -10°C [45]. Research of ionized calcium determination in turkeys revealed that there was no significant difference in ionized calcium levels in fresh plasma or serum. Sodium heparin was the most suitable anticoagulant. Ionized calcium in the serum and plasma stored at 4°C for 4 or 8 hours was significantly lower than in fresh samples [46]. In studies investigating ionized calcium levels in Thick-billed parrots (*Rhynchopsitta pachyrhyncha*) and Humboldt penguins (*Sphenicus humboldti*), ionized calcium was evaluated in frozen serum with no additional care to prevent contact with air in the tubes. The ionized calcium results were corrected to a standard pH of 7.4 using a regression formula developed for canine samples [47,48].

Ionized calcium determination is routinely done using analyzers with calcium ion-selective electrodes. Portable clinical analyzers, such as the i-STAT, allow immediate analysis of ionized calcium, minimizing the effects of sample storage in the results. Portable clinical analyzers can be used for ionized calcium determination in birds but their algorithms may not be validated for all species of birds. The tendency of this portable analyzer to underestimate ionized calcium greater than 1.3 mmol/L could also be a limitation, since most avian species studied have ionized calcium levels above that [49]. A recent study in chickens compared ionized calcium determination using i-STAT portable chemical analyzer to laboratory analyzer, with a good reliability and accuracy of results [50].

Ionized calcium levels have been determined for a few bird species (Table 3). In healthy animals, ionized calcium is tightly maintained within a narrow normal range, which is highly conserved within a given species [42]. Normal values should be established for each laboratory on the basis of species, type of sample, and analyzer used [2].

Vitamin D₃

Vitamin D_3 assays can be important in the evaluation of calcium disorders, especially when related to hypo- or hypervitaminosis D. Vitamin D_3 levels in birds are best assessed by evaluation the concentration of 25-OH-D_3 in the blood since this vitamin D metabolite is the most abundant and has a longer half life [15,51]. The metabolites of vitamin D are chemically identical in all species so assays used in humans are satisfactory for use in animals [2]. There are two available commercial assays: radioimmunoassay (RIA for 25-OH-D_3 and 1,25-$(OH)_2$-D_3) and enzyme immunoassay (EIA for 25-OH-D_3). RIA was used in American crows for diagnosis of nutritional secondary hyperparathyroidism in free-living birds [52] and for the determination of normal blood levels of 25-OH-D_3 in captive Thick-billed parrots [47] and Humboldt penguins [48]. EIA was used for measurement of 25-OH-D_3 in healthy African gray parrots [53].

Blood should be drawn into heparin and plasma frozen immediately until the assay can be performed [4]. Avoid exposure to light for long periods [2].

Any results for 25-OH-D_3 determination should be interpreted within the context of the diet, reproductive activity, and UV-B light exposure [4]. Vitamin D concentration in domestic chicken is dramatically affected by sampling time in relation to reproductive status and stage of eggshell

Table 3

Reference range of blood levels of ionized calcium, 25-OH-D_3 and PTH in different avian species

Species	iCa (mmol/L)	25-D₃ (nmol/L)	PTH (pmol/L)
Blue and gold macaw [54]	1.15–1.55		
Domestic chicken [1,42]	1.3–1.6	27.2–68	0.05–0.5[e]
Thick-billed parrot [47]	0.82–1.3[a]	5.2–51[c]	0–65.68
Caribbean flamingo [49]	1.3–1.4[b]		
African gray parrot [53]	0.96–1.2[a]	7.2–380[d]	
Humboldt penguin [48]	1.19–1.39[a]	1.3–6.1[c]	0.5–1.1
	1.12–1.3 [b]		
American crow [52]		13.6–26.4[c]	
Silver king pigeon [52]		30.8–35[c]	
Ostrich [8]			203–207

[a] Laboratory analyzer.
[b] Portable chemical analyzer.
[c] Radioimmunoassay.
[d] Enzyme immunoassay.
[e] Levels of PTH-like activity for egg-laying birds.

calcification [1]. Table 3 presents normal 25-OH-D_3 values for some bird species.

PTH

Few reports exist of blood concentrations of PTH in birds, likely reflecting that they are normally very low and, until recently, pure avian PTH was not available for antibody production [1]. In mammals, PTH assays are used for diagnosis of primary and secondary hyperparathyroidism and malignant hypercalcemia.

Parathyroid hormone assay is very labile, requiring precise sample handling to produce good results. Blood should be collected into EDTA and assayed immediately or frozen at $-70°C$ within 1 hour of collecting the sample. Serum is also adequate if stored frozen after separation from blood [2,4].

Only intact PTH is biologically active and it is best to measure this form. Because of the very short life of the biologically active 1 to 34 section, most human assays concentrate on the whole PTH molecule or on the middle and terminal segments [2]. Since the segment with most similarity between birds and mammals is the initial 1 to 34 section, the use of these mammalian assays could potentially be limited. A recent study investigated the use of a human research kit for 1 to 34 N section PTH in African gray parrots, with consistent results [55]. This test is difficult to use routinely and commercial assays are no longer available [4,55]. Intact 1 to 84 PTH human assays are not useful in psittacine birds [4]. A mid-molecule PTH (44 to 68)-based commercial RIA kit designed for use in humans has been used successfully for determination of PTH concentration in ostriches [8] and Thick-billed parrots [47]. In a study with Humboldt penguins, a standard mammalian sandwich procedure for intact PTH was used [48]. PTH-like activity has been determined in chickens during the egg-laying cycle, with levels being higher during the phase of eggshell calcification (inverse relationship with ionized calcium levels) [1]. The correlation between PTH-like and PTH has not been established in birds [47].

Serum PTH concentrations should always be evaluated in relationship to simultaneous measurement of serum total or ionized calcium concentration. If the parathyroid glands are normal, hypercalcemia should be associated with low PTH concentration, whereas a high PTH concentration should occur during hypocalcemia [2]. Also, PTH is reported to vary widely during the day, requiring multiple samples for accurate evaluation of PTH status [1]. Table 3 presents normal PTH and PTH-like activity levels for different species of birds.

No standards of PTH determination in birds have been established. Further investigation of intact mammalian PTH assay or any other assay in avian species is warranted before the usefulness and validation of these tests can be determined.

Common calcium metabolism disorders

Calcium deficiency/hypocalcemia

Table 2 presents causes of hypocalcemia in birds. The most common cause of calcium deficiency/hypocalcemia in birds is dietary, either from deficiency in calcium, phosphorus, or vitamin D_3 or diets that contain an inadequate calcium:phosphorus (Ca:P) ratio. Lack of exposure to UV-B light can also affect calcium bioavailability because of decreased production of vitamin D_3. Excessive dietary manganese also prevents normal absorption of intestinal calcium [56].

Grains and seeds commonly fed to psittacine birds have low calcium levels, low to none vitamin D_3, excess phosphorus, and excess fat. High levels of phosphorus and fat will reduce bioavailability of calcium in the diet because of the formation of complexes in the intestine [3,35,56]. Carnivorous birds fed an all-meat diet (Ca:P ratio 1:20), day-old chicks, or pinky mice receive a diet deficient in calcium and with excessive phosphorus [57]. This is also a concern for insect-eating birds in captivity, since most invertebrates have an abnormal calcium-phosphorus ratio [28].

Hypovitaminosis D_3 mimics calcium deficiency because of the important role of this vitamin in calcium homeostasis. Vitamin D_3 deficiency can be secondary to (1) decreased dietary intake; (2) decreased absorption as a result of intestinal disorders; or (3) decreased production because of reduced exposure to direct UV-B light or primary disease of the liver or kidney [34].

Other causes of hypocalcemia in mammals, such as primary hypoparathyroidism, pseudohypoparathyroidism, renal secondary hyperparathyroidism, intestinal malabsorption, and severe rhabdomyolysis (as a cause of hypocalcemia), have not been reported in birds [58,59]. Although hypocalcemia can occur in cases of renal failure, there has been no definitive correlation between electrolyte abnormalities and renal disease in birds [6,30].

With persistent low intestinal uptake of calcium, the parathyroid gland is constantly stimulated to release PTH in an effort to maintain blood calcium concentrations. This results in parathyroid hyperplasia (secondary nutritional hyperparathyroidism) and excessive bone mobilization. The resorbed bone is replaced by fibrous connective tissue. Because calcium is very important to the organism, blood calcium levels are preserved and hypocalcemia is not detected until bone reserves are severely depleted [59].

Nutritional secondary hyperparathyroidism (NSH) has been reported in numerous species of captive birds [56,60]. Results of a retrospective study of parathyroid gland lesions in birds revealed that over 80% of the cases of parathyroid hyperplasia involved psittacine birds, with African gray parrots being the species with higher incidence (37.5%) [61]. NSH is rare in free-living birds and, to the author's knowledge, has only been reported in wild fledgling American crows (*Corvus brachyrhynchus brachyrhynchus*) in Northeast United States [52], in nestling Cattle egrets (*Bubulcus ibis*) in Texas [62], and in nestling Cape vultures (*Gyps coprotheres*) in South Africa

[63]. Bone deformities associated with calcium deficiency have been reported in Great tits (*Parus major*), Black terns (*Chlidonias niger*), and White storks (*Ciconia ciconia*) in Europe, presumptively related with soil acidification and consequent reduced levels of calcium in soil, plants, and ingested prey [64,65].

The various conditions that occur as a result of calcium deficiency and associated hyperparathyroidism are often referred to as metabolic bone disease, which includes the various forms of rickets seen in young growing birds, osteomalacia in adult birds, and osteoporosis, also known as caged layer fatigue [58].

Clinical signs of calcium deficiency vary with species, age, sex, gender, reproductive status, and degree of deficiency. In the early stages, adult female birds commonly present with abnormal eggs (soft, misshaped, thin shell), egg binding, and poor reproductive performance (mainly because of increased embryo mortality); osteomalacia with pathological fractures and "cage paralysis" will develop with persistent calcium deficiency. Adult birds can also present bone deformities and poor feather condition with feather picking. Growing birds can present with abnormal growth, skeletal deformities, or fractures in the long bones and/or spinal column (with secondary paralysis). Neurological signs, ranging from weakness and ataxia to seizures, develop in the more advanced stages of the disease when calcium blood levels are low and are more frequently seen in African gray parrots [4,8,56].

Diagnosis is based on history of a poor diet and/or increased calcium demand (growth, egg laying), physical exam findings, radiographs, and blood chemistries. Radiographs of affected birds can reveal poor bone mineralization, pathological fractures, and/or bone deformities (Fig. 4) [31,56]. In

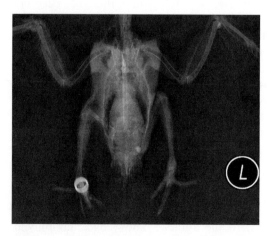

Fig. 4. Ventrodorsal radiograph of an adult female cockatiel with a 7-day history of anorexia, lethargy, and lameness. This bird was offered an all-seed diet. The overall bone density is reduced and the right radius and ulna and left tarsometatarus present pathological fractures. The plasma total calcium levels in this bird were within reference range for the species.

most cases, alkaline phosphatase levels are elevated and total blood calcium levels are normal or elevated, both as a result of increased PTH activity in response to lower bioavailability of calcium [56]. Measurement of PTH blood levels could potentially aid the diagnosis of NSH. Response of a convulsing bird to a calcium injection is also diagnostic [31].

Hypocalcemic seizures occur frequently in adult African gray parrots. The syndrome could potentially be classified as nutritional secondary hyperparathyroidism because, in general, affected birds are offered diets deficient in calcium and vitamin D (all seed diets) and parathyroid hyperplasia is observed on necropsy. Despite this, radiographic appearance and histopathology of the skeleton is normal, and plasma alkaline phosphatase levels are within reference range, suggesting an osteoclast dysfunction and impaired calcium immobilization from the bone. When dietary calcium and vitamin D are limited, bioavailability of calcium is low and since bone resorption appears to be impaired, birds will develop hypocalcemia and secondary neurological signs. The incidence of this syndrome appears to be decreasing with improvement of feeding practices. It has been demonstrated that African gray parrots have lower concentrations of calcium, total protein, and albumin when compared with Amazon parrots, which could also contribute to the higher incidence of this problem in African gray parrots [35]. There has been also some undocumented discussion that the syndrome is limited to imported birds and is more common on the West Coast as compared with the East Coast of the United States [57,59]. Hypocalcemic tetany has been also reported in a Green-cheeked Amazon parrot [66].

Treatment in acute cases consists of injectable calcium gluconate (10 to 100 mg/kg intramuscularly), together with supportive care. Exercise restriction and careful handling and restraint are necessary to avoid development of pathological fractures. To aid treatment and prevent recurrence, the diet needs to be adjusted to the recommended levels of calcium, phosphorus, and vitamin D_3 for the age and species.

Prognosis of calcium deficiency for young and adult birds will depend on severity of bone abnormalities and other clinical conditions that may develop.

Excessive calcium/hypercalcemia

Causes of hypocalcemia in birds are presented in Table 2. Hypercalcemia in birds is most often physiologic and associated with increased estrogen secretion and production of calcium-binding proteins. Total calcium in these birds can be as high as 40 mg/dL without clinical complications. Pathological hypercalcemia in birds is most commonly secondary to marked and prolonged excessive dietary calcium and/or vitamin D_3. Other causes of hypercalcemia in mammals, such as primary hyperparathyroidism, pseudohyperparathyroidism (hypercalcemia associated with neoplasia), and cholecalciferol rodenticide ingestion have not been reported in birds [5,59].

Hypercalcinosis secondary to prolonged excessive dietary calcium has been described in chickens, ostriches, and budgerigars. In a study involving budgerigars, increasing levels of dietary calcium were showed to be more toxic to the kidneys than hypervitaminosis D_3. In this same study, birds had lesions consistent with calcium toxicosis with calcium concentrations in the diet as low as 0.7% [30].

Hypervitaminosis D_3 will cause an excessive calcium uptake from the intestine and mimic hypercalcinosis. Vitamin D toxicity is exacerbated by high dietary levels of either calcium or phosphorus. The relative toxicity of the vitamin D metabolites follows the same pattern as their bioactivity: $D_2 < D_3 < 25$-OH-$D_3 < 1,25$-$(OH)_2$-D_3 [16]. Little information is known about required and toxic levels of vitamin D for most avian species. In poultry, it appears that at least 100 times the recommended dose can be tolerated. Some authors suggest that toxicity can occur as low as 4 to 10 times the recommended dose [30]. Different species appear to have different needs and sensitivities to vitamin D_3, as observed with the higher incidence of vitamin D toxicity in macaws, especially Blue and Gold and Hyacinth macaws [34]. Cockatiels have also been noted to be particularly sensitive to high calcium and/or vitamin D_3 levels in the diet [57]. Another species that appears to be susceptible to hypervitaminosis D_3 is the African gray parrot, although any species of bird can be affected [30].

Most cases of calcium and vitamin D_3 toxicosis have been described in growing psittacine birds associated with feeding commercial diets supplemented with a mineral and/or vitamin supplement, raising the calcium and/or vitamin D content of the diet to toxic levels [30,34,67]. Long-term consumption of high levels of calcium may interfere also with magnesium, manganese, and zinc absorption, causing secondary deficiencies [3].

As a result of hypercalcinosis, calcification of soft tissues (including arterial walls), nephrocalcinosis, visceral gout, and urate nephrosis can develop. Clinical signs include poor weight gain and hatchability, increased embryo mortality (toxic levels of calcium and vitamin D_3 are transferred to the embryo), depression, anorexia, nausea, polyuria and polydipsia, painful joints, and muscle weakness [28–30,59].

Diagnosis is based on thorough dietary history, radiographs, and blood testing. Calcification of soft tissues and renomegaly can be observed on radiographs. Routine blood chemistry abnormalities include hyperuricemia and hypercalcemia, although this condition should not be ruled out in eucalcemic patients. Measurement of vitamin D_3 metabolites in the blood could potentially aid the diagnosis of hypervitaminosis D_3. In normal birds experimentally subject to hypervitaminosis D, 25-OH-D_3 and not 1,25-$(OH)_2$-D_3, was increased in the serum [30].

Treatment includes diuresis with a calcium-deficient crystalloid, such as NaCl 0.9% and diet correction. Furosemide treatment is recommended for cases of persistent hypercalcemia following diuresis with crystalloid fluids. In mammals, treatment with calcitonin is advocated for cases of severe and/or persistent hypercalcemia, as calcitonin rapidly decreases the magnitude of hypercalcemia [2,59]. There have been no reports of the clinical use of calcitonin in birds [59].

Prognosis of hypercalcinosis is poor if tissue calcification and visceral or articular gout are present.

Summary

Calcium concentration in the blood is controlled by many interacting feedback loops that involve calcium, phosphate, PTH, vitamin D_3, and calcitonin. In egg-laying birds, sex hormones also contribute to calcium homeostasis. These mechanisms help maintain blood concentration of calcium in a narrow range for normal function of the body. Calcium metabolism disorders are common in birds, mainly metabolic bone disease and hypercalcinosis secondary to excess of calcium and/or vitamin D_3 in the diet. Complete history (including diet), physical examination, routine blood tests, and imaging may aid diagnosis. Determination of ionized calcium has proven to be an important tool in investigating calcium disorders in birds, especially in cases where blood concentrations of proteins are abnormal. Although blood concentration of vitamin D_3 and PTH in some avian species has been determined, more research needs to be done to validate assays and results until these tests can be used for diagnostic purposes.

Acknowledgments

The author thanks Dr. James Morrisey for his mentorship and help in preparation of this article.

References

[1] Dacke CG. The parathyroids, calcitonin, and vitamin D. In: Wittow GC, editor. Sturkie's Avian Physiology. 5th edition. Orlando (FL): Academic Press; 2000. p. 473–88.
[2] Rosol TJ, Chew DJ, Nagode LA, et al. Disorders of calcium: hypercalcemia and hypocalcemia. In: DiBartola SP, editor. Fluid therapy in small animal clinical practice. 2nd edition. Philadelphia: WB Saunders; 2000. p. 108–61.
[3] Klansing KC. Minerals. In: Comparative avian nutrition. New York: CAB International; 1998. p. 234–75.
[4] Stanford M. Calcium metabolism. In: Harrison GJ, Lightfoot TL, editors. Clinical avian medicine, vol 1Palm Beach (FL): Spix Publishing; 2006. p. 141–51.
[5] Jones MP. Avian clinical pathology. Vet Clin North Am Exot Anim Pract 1999;2(3):663–88.
[6] Taylor TG, Dacke CG. Calcium metabolism and its regulation. In: Freeman BM, editor. Physiology and biochemistry of the domestic fowl, vol. 5Orlando (FL): Academic Press; 1984. p. 125–70.
[7] King AS, McLelland J. Endocrine system. In: Birds, their structure and function. 2nd edition. Philadelphia: Bailliere Tindall; 1984. p. 200–13.
[8] Yagil R, van Creveld C, Levy A. Ostrich endocrinology II: PTH and calcium. International Journal of Animal Science 1993;8:5–8.
[9] Kenny AD. Parathyroid and ultimobranchial glands. In: Sturkie PD, editor. Avian physiology. 4th edition. New York: Springer-Verlag; 1986. p. 466–78.
[10] Lasmoles F, Jullienne A, Desplan C, et al. Structure of chicken calcitonin predicted by partial nucleotide sequence of its precursor. FEBS Lett 1985;180(1):113–6.

[11] Kapoor AS, Chhabra SK. Relative physiological activity of calcitonin in the thyroid and ultimobranchial glands of the pigeon, *Columbia livia Gmelin*. Gen Comp Endocrinol 1981; 44:307–13.

[12] Norman AW, Hurwitz S. The role of the vitamin D endocrine system in avian bone biology. J Nutr 1993;123(Suppl 2):310–6.

[13] Yasuoka T, Kawashima M, Takahashi T, et al. Calcitonin receptor binding properties in bone and kidney of the chicken during the oviposition cycle. J Bone Miner Res 1998; 13(9):1412–9.

[14] Rasmussen H, Wong M, Bickle D. Hormonal control of the renal conversion of 25-hydroxycholecalciferol to 1,25-dihydroxycholecalciferol. J Clin Invest 1972;51:2502–4.

[15] Norman AW. Studies of the vitamin D endocrine system in the avian. J Nutr 1987;117(4): 797–807.

[16] Klasing KC. Vitamins. In: Comparative avian nutrition. New York: CAB International; 1998. p. 277–329.

[17] Aslam SM, Garlich JD, Qureshi MA. Vitamin D deficiency alters the immune response of broiler chicks. Poult Sci 1998;77(6):842–9.

[18] Trump DL, Hershberger PA, Bernardi RJ, et al. Anti-tumor activity of calcitriol: pre-clinical and clinical studies. J Steroid Biochem Mol Biol 2004;89–90:519–26.

[19] Tian XQ, Chen TC, Zhiren L, et al. Characterization of the translocation process of vitamin D3 from the skin into circulation. Endocrinology 1994;135(2):655–61.

[20] Johnson AL. Reproduction in the female. In: Wittow GC, editor. Sturkie's avian physiology. 5th edition. Orlando (FL): Academic Press; 2000. p. 569–96.

[21] Klasing KC. Avian macrophages: regulators of local and systemic immune responses. Poult Sci 1998;77:938–89.

[22] Whitehead CC. Overview of bone biology in the egg-laying hen. Poult Sci 2004;83:193–9.

[23] Shaw AJ, Dacke CG. Cyclic nucleotides and the rapid inhibitions of bone 45Ca uptake in response to bovine parathyroid hormone and 16,16-dimethyl prostaglandin E2 in chicks. Calcif Tissue Int 1989;44:209–13.

[24] Joyner KL. Theriogenology. In: Ritchie BW, Harrison GJ, Harrison LR, editors. Avian medicine: principles and aplication. Lake Worth (FL): Wingers; 1994. p. 749–804.

[25] Baski SN, Kenny AD. Vitamin D metabolism in Japanese quail: gonadal hormones and dietary calcium effects. Am J Physiol 1978;234(6):E622–8.

[26] Beck MM, Hansen KK. Role of estrogen in avian osteoporosis. Poult Sci 2004;83:200–6.

[27] Koutsos EA, Matson KD, Klasing KC. Nutrition of birds in the order Psittaciformes: a review. Journal of Avian Medicine and Surgery 2001;15(4):257–75.

[28] McDonald D. Nutrition and dietary supplementation. In: Harrison GJ, Lightfoot TL, editors. Clinical avian medicine, vol. 1Palm Beach (FL): Spix Publishing; 2006. p. 86–107.

[29] Roudybush TE. Psittacine nutrition. Vet Clin North Am Exot Anim Pract 1999;2(1):111–26.

[30] Echols MS. Evaluating and treating the kidney. In: Harrison GJ, Lightfoot TL, editors. Clinical avian medicine, vol. 2Palm Beach (FL): Spix Publishing; 2006. p. 451–91.

[31] Smith JM, Roudybush TE. Nutritional disorders. In: Altman RB, Clubb SL, Dorrestein GD, Quesenberry K, editors. Avian medicine and surgery. Philadelphia: Saunders; 1997. p. 501–15.

[32] Stanford M. The effect of UV-B lighting supplementation in African grey parrots. Exotic DVM 2004;6(3):29–32.

[33] Atencio A, Edwards HM Jr, Pesti GM, et al. The vitamin D3 requirements of broiler breeders. Poult Sci 2006;85(4):674–92.

[34] Roudybush T. Nutritional disorders. In: Rosskopf WJ, Woerpel RW, editors. Diseases of caged and aviary birds. Baltimore (MD): Williams and Wilkins; 1996. p. 490–500.

[35] Goodman GJ. Metabolic disorders. In: Rosskopf WJ, Woerpel RW, editors. Diseases of caged and aviary birds. Baltimore (MD): Williams and Wilkins; 1996. p. 470–8.

[36] Fudge AM. Avian metabolic disorders. In: Fudge AM, editor. Laboratory medicine: avian and exotic pets. Philadelphia: WB Saunders; 2000. p. 56–60.

[37] Schenck PA, Chew DJ. Prediction of serum ionized calcium concentration by use of serum total calcium concentration in dogs. Am J Vet Res 2005;66(8):1330–6.

[38] Lumeij JT. Relation of plasma calcium to total protein and albumin in African grey (*Psittacus erithacus*) and Amazon (*Amazona* spp.) parrots. Avian Pathol 1900;661–7.

[39] Stanford MD. Measurement of ionized calcium in grey parrots: the effect of diet. In: Proc 7th Euro Assoc Avian Vet Conference. Tenerife, Spain: 2003.

[40] Lumeij JT, Remple JD, Riddle KE. Relationship of plasma total protein and albumin to total calcium in peregrine falcons (*Falco peregrinus*). Avian Pathol 1993;22:183–8.

[41] Verstappen ALM, Lumeij JT, Bronneberg RGG. Plasma chemistry reference values in ostriches. J Wildl Dis 2002;38(1):154–9.

[42] Harr KE. Clinical chemistry of companion avian species: a review. Vet Clin Pathol 2002;31: 140–51.

[43] Luck MR. The measurement of ionized calcium concentration in chicken plasma during eggshell formation and in paired samples of fetal and maternal ovine plasma. J Physiol 1979;290(2):1P–2P.

[44] Parsons AH, Combs GF. Blood ionized calcium cycles in the chicken. Poult Sci 1981;60(7): 1520–4.

[45] Schenck PA, Chew DJ, Brooks CL. Effects of storage on serum ionized calcium and pH values in clinically normal dogs. Am J Vet Res 1995;56(3):304–7.

[46] McMurtry JP, Rosenbrough RW, Steele NC. Studies on blood calcium relationships in the turkey. Poult Sci 1984;63(10):2094–9.

[47] Howard LL, Kass PH, Lamberski N, et al. Serum concentrations of ionized calcium, vitamin D3 and parathyroid hormone in captive thick-billed parrots (*Rhynchopsitta pachyrhyncha*). J Zoo Wildl Med 2004;35(2):147–53.

[48] Adkesson MJ, Langan JN. Metabolic bone disease in juvenile Humboldt penguins (*Spheniscus humboldti*): investigation of ionized calcium, parathyroid hormone, and vitamin D3 as diagnostic parameters. J Zoo Wildl Med 2007;38(1):85–92.

[49] Howard LL. Preliminary use and literature review of the I-STAT (a portable clinical analyzer) in birds. In: Proc Am Assoc Zoo Vet Conference. Milwaukee: 2002. p. 96–100.

[50] Steinmetz HW, Vogt R, Kastner S, et al. Evaluation of the i-STAT portable clinical analyzer in chickens (*Gallus gallus*). J Vet Diagn Invest 2007;19(4):382–8.

[51] Stanford MD. Measurement of 25-hydroxycholecalciferol in grey parrots (*Psittacus e erithacus*). Vet Rec 2003;153:58–61.

[52] Tangredi BP, Krook LP. Nutritional secondary hyperparathyroidism in free-living fledgling American crows (*Corvus brachyrhynchos brachyrhynchos*). J Zoo Wildl Med 1999;30(1): 94–9.

[53] Stanford MD. Calcium metabolism in grey parrots: the effects of husbandry. Available at: http://www.hbf-uk.co.uk/downloads/stanford-calcium.pdf. Accessed June 1, 2007.

[54] Raphael BL. Hematology and blood chemistries of macaws. Proc Am Assoc Zoo Vet Conference. Washington DC: 1980. p. 97–8.

[55] Rosol TJ, Chew DJ, Nagode LA, et al. Pathophysiology of calcium metabolism. Vet Clin Pathol 1995;24(2):49–63.

[56] Wallach JD, Flieg GM. Nutritional secondary hyperparathyroidism in captive birds. J Am Vet Med Assoc 1969;155(7):1046–51.

[57] Macwhirter P. Malnutrition. In: Ritchie BW, Harrison GJ, Harrison LR, editors. Avian medicine: principles and application. Lake Worth (FL): Wingers; 1994. p. 842–61.

[58] Rae M. Avian endocrine disorders. In: Fudge AM, editor. Laboratory medicine: avian and exotic pets. Philadelphia: WB Saunders; 2000. p. 76–89.

[59] Johnston MS, Ivey ES. Parathyroid and ultimobranchial glands: calcium metabolism in birds. Seminars in Avian and Exotic Pet Medicine 2002;11(2):84–93.

[60] Folwer ME. Metabolic bone disease. In: Fowler ME, editor. Zoo and wildlife animal medicine. 2nd edition. Philadelphia: W.B. Saunders; 1986. p. 70–89.

[61] Schimdt RE, Reavill DR. Endocrine lesions in Psittacine birds. Proceedings AAV Conference. San Antonio: 2006. p. 27–9.
[62] Phalen DN, Drew ML, Contreras C, et al. Naturally occurring secondary nutritional hyperparathyroidism in cattle egrets (*Bubulcus ibis*) from central Texas. J Wildl Dis 2005;41(2): 401–15.
[63] Evans LB, Piper S. Bone abnormalities in the Cape vulture (*Gyps coprotheres*). J S Afr Vet Assoc 1981;52:67–8.
[64] Graveland J. Calcium deficiency in wild birds. Vet Q 1996;18(Suppl 3):S136–7.
[65] Smits JE, Bortolotti GR, Baos R, et al. Disrupted bone metabolism in contaminant-exposed white storks (*Ciconia ciconia*) in southwestern Spain. Environ Pollut 2007;145:538–44.
[66] Randell MG. Nutritionally induced hypocalcemic tetany in an Amazon parrot. J Am Vet Med Assoc 1981;179:1277–8.
[67] Schoemaker NJ, Lumeij JT, Beynen AC. Polyuria and polydipsia due to vitamin and mineral oversupplementation of the diet of a salmon crested cockatoo (*Cacatua moluccensis*) and blue and gold macaw (*Ara ararauna*). Avian Pathol 1997;26:201–9.

ELSEVIER
SAUNDERS

VETERINARY
CLINICS
Exotic Animal Practice

Vet Clin Exot Anim 11 (2008) 83–105

Update on Neuroendocrine Regulation and Medical Intervention of Reproduction in Birds

Christoph Mans, Med Vet*, W. Michael Taylor, DVM

Avian and Exotic Animal Service, Veterinary Teaching Hospital, Ontario Veterinary College, University of Guelph, College Avenue, Guelph, Ontario N1G 2W1, Canada

Every clinician treating birds is confronted with patients suffering from pathology caused by abnormalities of the neuroendocrine system controlling reproduction. Common presentations such as chronic egg laying, dystocia, cloacal and oviductal prolapse, undesirable behaviors (eg, aggression, feather plucking, self-mutilation), and reproductive misbehavior (eg, masturbation, excessive nesting) may reflect abnormalities in this system. Current medical treatment options for these conditions are often disappointing. A possible reason for these poor outcomes is the lack of knowledge of the underlying neuroendocrine, behavioral, and autonomous physiology of reproductive processes in avian species. Tremendous progress has been made over the last few years in our understanding of the neuroendocrine control of reproduction in birds. A hypothalamic gonadotropin-inhibiting hormone (GnIH) has been discovered, information on the role of melatonin and its influence on avian reproduction has grown, and the structure of avian GnRH and its receptors has been defined and compared with their mammalian counterparts.

In order to develop appropriate and safe treatment protocols for avian patients suffering from disorders related to the reproductive system, advantage should be taken of these experimentally derived data.

This article attempts neither to review the vast amount of literature on the role of neuroendocrine physiology of reproduction in birds nor to provide a complete review of avian reproductive physiology and endocrinology, because such articles have been published previously [1–8]. The intent of this article is to focus on the current exciting discoveries and new opinions in avian reproductive neuroendocrinology and their possible applications to clinical avian medicine.

---

* Corresponding author.
E-mail address: cmans@gmx.net (C. Mans).

1094-9194/08/$ - see front matter © 2008 Elsevier Inc. All rights reserved.
doi:10.1016/j.cvex.2007.09.003

Hormones of the hypothalamus

The hypothalamic control of gonadotropins secreted from the anterior pituitary gland (eg, luteinizing hormone [LH], follicle-stimulating hormone [FSH], prolactin) is regulated by neuropeptides and neurotransmitters released from the median eminence and transported by the hypophyseal portal vascular system to the anterior pituitary gland [9].

GnRH

In birds, as in other vertebrates, the hypothalamic decapeptide GnRH is the primary factor responsible for the hypothalamic control of gonadotropin secretion [10,11]. GnRH plays a key role in the control of sexual maturity, ovulation rate, semen production, incubation, photorefractoriness, and reproductive aging, which all appear to be related to alterations in GnRH regulation [12]. Some investigators prefer to use the term "luteinizing hormone-releasing hormone," because only the ability to control directly the release of the gonadotropin LH in vivo and not FSH has been demonstrated clearly in avian species [13,14]. Although GnRH may not directly stimulate FSH release in vivo, it may have an indirect effect by controlling FSH synthesis [15]. Other factors, such as gonadal steroids and gonadal peptide hormones such as inhibin, may play a more significant role in avian FSH synthesis and release control than GnRH [12].

Three forms of GnRH have been identified in birds: chicken GnRH-I (cGnRH-I) [16], chicken GnRH-II (cGnRH-II) [17], and lamprey GnRH-III (lGnRH-III) [18]. Although cGnRH-I and -II were first described in the chicken, they have also been found in all avian species so far investigated. lGnRH-III has been detected in the hypothalamus and forebrain of house sparrows (*Passer domesticus*) and white-crowned sparrows (*Zonotrichia leucophrys gambelii*) [18]. lGnRH-III has a widespread distribution throughout the central nervous system of investigated passerine species, with particular focal concentration in auditory processing and song-producing areas. Furthermore, lGnRH-III has gonadotropin-releasing capabilities in vivo. Auditory processing, song production, and the influence of gonadotropin release may be directly linked in song birds [18].

cGnRH-I and -II have distinctly different distributions in the avian nervous system, and therefore, different functions. Most cGnRH-I cell bodies are found predominately in the hypothalamus, but numerous extrahypothalamic sites have been reported [12,15,19–21]. cGnRH-I terminals are found in large quantities in the median eminence, as expected for a neuroendocrine hormone that enters the hypophyseal portal vasculature to control anterior pituitary function [12,15,22]. In contrast, the presence of cGnRH-II terminals in the median eminence remains controversial. Although several immunohistologic studies have demonstrated the absence of cGnRH-II in the median eminence [21,23], two studies have demonstrated that the median eminence of Japanese quail (*Coturnix japonica*) and domestic chicken contain cGnRH-II immunoreactive peptides [24,25]. cGnRH-II cell bodies are found in low amounts scattered throughout the brain. Several predominant locations (eg, the region of the juncture of the diencephalon and mesencephalon and the caudal basal hypothalamus) have been described [12,15,21].

Although the physiologic function of cGnRH-I is predominantly the direct control of LH release from the anterior pituitary gland, the function of GnRH-II remains unclear. Active immunization against cGnRH-I, but not against cGnRH-II, in chickens resulted in complete suppression of egg production and a decrease in plasma LH concentration, in contrast to repeated active immunization against cGnRH-II, which had no impact on egg production or plasma LH concentration [21].

The preovulatory release of LH in chicken is accompanied by a decrease of cGnRH-I, whereas hypothalamic cGnRH-II concentrations are unchanged [26]. In contrast, ovariectomy in the turkey caused significant reductions in cGnRH-I and -II concentrations of the hypothalamus [27]. In young male chickens, hypothalamic GnRH-I concentrations, not cGnRH-II, are increased at the onset of puberty [21]. Although cGnRH-II has a more potent effect than cGnRH-I on LH release in vitro, the current data provide no strong evidence for direct involvement of cGnRH-II in vivo in the release of LH and it is therefore believed to be nonhypophysiotropic [28]. Instead, an important role in female sexual behavior, independent of cGnRH-I, has been suggested [28]. Intracerebroventricular injections of GnRH-II, but not of GnRH-I, enhanced courtship behavior in estrogen-primed female white-crowed sparrows (*Zonotrichia leucophrys gambelii*) [28].

Changes in the concentration of hypothalamic cGnRH-I and -II have been shown to be related to several factors that differ, depending on the species. In turkeys, hypothalamic cGnRH-I concentrations were highest in laying hens, followed by photostimulated and incubating birds. The lowest hypothalamic cGnRH-I concentrations were measured in nonlaying hens. Hypothalamic cGnRH-II concentrations were highest after photostimulation and returned to nonphotostimulated levels during incubation and photorefractoriness [27].

Two different cGnRH receptors (cGnRHR-I, cGnRHR-II) and several splice variants have been identified [29]. Receptor expression, affinity, and responsiveness appear to depend on the reproductive stage and age [11]. Although levels of cGnRHR-I remain constant between reproductive stages in chickens, the pituitary levels of cGnRHR-II mRNA are directly correlated with the reproductive status [11]. Most of the different cGnRH forms can bind and activate every cGnRHR, but differences in affinity and specificity are reported [11,30].

Gonadotropin-inhibiting hormone

Until recently, it was widely accepted that vertebrates had no gonadotropin-inhibiting factor of hypothalamic origin, and the only inhibiting factors on gonadotropin release were thought to be gonadal sex steroids and inhibin by negative feedback mechanism [10]. However, in the year 2000, a hypothalamic dodecapeptide, which directly acts on the pituitary to inhibit gonadotropin release, was first described in Japanese quail (*Coturnix japonica*) and was termed GnIH [31].

GnIH cell bodies and terminals are predominately located in the median eminence and the paraventricular nucleus of the hypothalamus [10]. GnIH receptors are expressed in the pituitary gland and several brain regions, including the hypothalamus [10]. GnIH acts directly on the pituitary by way of GnIH receptors [10]. A direct contact between GnIH axon terminals and GnRH-I and -II neurons was recently discovered as well as the expression of GnIH receptor mRNA in GnRH-I and -II neurons [32]. Therefore, it is suspected that GnIH may additionally directly inhibit GnRH release from the hypothalamus into the portal blood system [10,32,33]. Moreover, other regions of the central nervous system, including the cerebrum, mesencephalon, and spinal cord contain GnIH receptor mRNA, suggestive of multiple as-yet-undefined regulatory functions of GnIH in the avian brain [34,35].

The control of GnIH has not been investigated extensively, but melatonin seems to play a key role in this function [36]. Pinealectomy combined with orbital enucleation decreased the expression of GnIH precursor mRNA and mature GnIH peptide expression in Japanese quail (*Coturnix japonica*). Melatonin administration in these birds resulted in a dose-dependent increase in GnIH mRNA and mature peptide expression [36]. Thus, GnIH may be capable of transducing photoperiodic information by way of changes in the melatonin signal to influence the reproductive axis of birds [10]. It has also been suggested that GnIH may play a primary role in timing the annual reproductive cycle in songbirds, specifically, the onset of photorefractoriness [33].

The functional significance of GnIH was demonstrated in several avian species, where administration led to decreased gonadotropin synthesis and secretion [10,37,38]. If GnIH was injected simultaneously with GnRH, it inhibited the rise of LH above baseline in song sparrows [38]. In mature male Japanese quail (*Coturnix japonica*), chronic administration of GnIH by way of osmotic pumps led to a decrease in plasma testosterone concentrations and gonadotropin synthesis and secretion, induced testicular apoptosis, and decreased spermatogenic activity in the testis. In immature male quail, normal testicular growth and testosterone levels were suppressed [37].

GnIH was found to stimulate feeding behavior in chicks and to inhibit female sexual behavior in white-crowned sparrows (*Zonotrichia leucophrys gambelii*) [35,39]. Therefore, GnIH may also play a role in behavior and autonomic mechanisms [10]. Because of the antagonistic actions of GnRH and GnIH on gonadotropin release, it is likely that they also act antagonistically on reproductive behavior, especially considering the distribution of GnIH fibers. If this turns out to be the case, then rapid activation or deactivation of the GnIH system could provide a mechanism by which the female songbirds respond correctly at a specific time of the year to social cues, and copulate with the appropriate partner (age, species) [35].

Hormones of the anterior pituitary gland

As in mammals, six different hormones (FSH, LH, prolactin, STH, ACTH, TSH) plus the melanotropic hormone are produced by the anterior pituitary gland (hypophysis) [5].

Although in mammals the gonadotropins LH and FSH are produced by the same subpopulation of cells and regulation is GnRH pulse frequency dependent, in avian species the two gonadotropins appear to be synthesized by two different cell types [40,41], which might be important because varying frequencies of pulsatile GnRH secretion in mammals differentially regulate LH and FSH synthesis and release during the ovarian cycle [11,42].

Follicle-stimulating hormone

FSH is a glycoprotein produced in the beta cells of the anterior pituitary gland [5]. In female birds, FSH is the key hormone for ovarian folliculogenesis and steroidogenesis. It is responsible for follicular maturation and differentiation, whereas ovulation results from a positive feedback mechanism caused by LH and progesterone [43]. FSH has influence on less mature, large, yolky follicles and small follicles, but not on large, preovulatory follicles [13]. FSH stimulates proliferation and differentiation of granulosa cells, stimulating progesterone and steroid hormone production [44]. In male birds, FSH not only stimulates tubular growth of the testes and spermatogenesis with the onset of puberty but also facilitates the long-term maintenance of quantitative normal spermatogenesis in mature male birds [5,44].

The control of FSH expression and release is not clearly understood in birds. In contrast to that in mammals, FSH does not seem to be controlled primarily by GnRH [13,44]. However, photostimulation, acting by way of the central nervous system, increases plasma FSH and pituitary FSH in chickens [14]. Moreover, estradiol and inhibin play a role in pituitary FSH secretion by way of negative feedback [44–46]. Other factors, such as activin and follistatin, may also play a role in FSH secretion [47]. Although it has been proposed that cGnRH-II or lGnRH-III may function as FSH-releasing hormones, no in vivo evidence exists to support this hypothesis [48]. Future research will show if there is a specific FSH-releasing factor, and therefore, this possibility should not be excluded.

FSH and LH are released in an asynchronous, pulsatile fashion [44,49]. The dynamic pulsatile pattern of FSH release seems necessary for the initiation and maintenance of spermatogenesis in the fowl [44].

Luteinizing hormone

In photoperiodic avian species, photoinduced LH secretion is generally associated with an increase in hypothalamic GnRH-I peptide [50]. The physiologic significance of GnRH-II on LH release is uncertain [51]. Several neurotransmitters, such as norepinephrine and epinephrine, have the potential to stimulate LH release, and others, such as dopamine, may inhibit release [51].

LH secretion reaches its peak levels 4 to 6 hours before ovulation in most investigated species [13]. With the onset of incubation, LH decreases; it may increase again after the young fledge in multiple-brooded species, but may not increase in single-brooded species because of the development of photo-refractoriness [9,51]. The seasonal maximum LH level in photoperiodic species precedes that of prolactin [51]. Removing eggs from an incubating female bird will result in an increase in LH secretion, which is associated with an increase of GnRH-I mRNA in the hypothalamus [52].

Injection of LH leads to an increase of plasma concentrations of progesterone, estrogens, and androgens, by stimulating their synthesis and release from the gonads [13]. In male birds, LH stimulates the Leydig cells to differentiate and produce testosterone [13].

Prolactin

Avian prolactin-producing cells (lactotrophs) are located in the anterior pituitary gland [53]. Prolactin receptors are widely distributed in the digestive, osmoregulatory, immune, reproductive, and neural systems, consistent with its known involvement in multiple physiologic processes [54].

The hypothalamic vasoactive intestinal polypeptide (VIP) is thought to be the major prolactin-releasing factor in avian species and regulates prolactin secretion by acting directly on the anterior pituitary gland [51,55,56]. Other factors, such as dopamine, 5-hydroxtryptophan, and the opioid peptide dynorphin, exert some central nervous effects on prolactin release [57–59]. Thyroxin administration can enhance prolactin secretion in starlings and induces photorefractoriness [60].

In many instances, it is not known if prolactin is a neuromodulatory agent that acts directly on the brain or if its effects are mediated through interactions with peripheral target organs, which, in turn, generate stimuli that promote neuromodulatory changes in the brain that can induce changes in incubation and parental behavior [61].

Prolactin has potent antigonadal and antigonadotropic effects [62,63]. It has been shown to suppress plasma LH in several avian species, although the response is not consistently observed in all studies [62–68]. Prolactin likely acts at the level of the hypothalamus and in the anterior pituitary gland to inhibit LH secretion [51,69]. Moreover, prolactin stimulates "crop milk" production related to the proliferation of mucosal cells of the ingluvies in columbiform species [13].

A positive feedback loop between prolactin and incubation is assumed and, in most species, the onset of incubation behavior is associated with increased prolactin secretion [51]. Circulating prolactin concentrations are elevated during the incubation of eggs and will decrease rapidly if incubation or nesting behavior is interrupted [65,70].

Tactile stimulation from eggs in the nest is an important factor for increasing prolactin secretion, which consequently increases incubation behavior [71–73]. The brood patch seems to be an important structure for receiving the tactile stimuli from the eggs. Local anesthesia of the brood patch for 9 hours caused a significant decrease in plasma prolactin concentrations in incubating female domestic ducks (*Anas platyrhynchos*) [73]. Turkey hens with denervated brood patches showed no increase in circulating prolactin levels after photostimulation, and no incubation behavior compared with the control group [71].

In photoperiodic species, the breeding season is terminated by an increase in prolactin secretion that leads to GnRH suppression after reaching a critical level of plasma prolactin [69]. If exogenous prolactin is administered systemically in female birds, it induces incubation behavior if it is preceded by nesting behavior and the attendant increases in plasma estrogens and progesterone [74]. In estrogen-primed female budgerigars (*Melopsittacus undulatus*), prolactin promotes extended nest-box occupation and incubation onset [75]. In ring doves (*Streptopelia risoria*), the onset of incubation appears to be induced by gonadal steroids alone, but systemically administered prolactin maintained readiness to incubate during long periods of separation from the nest and breeding partner, and extended the normal incubation period [76–78]. Systemically administered prolactin induces broody behavior toward chicks in gallinaceous species, and facilitates and increases the intensity of continued parental behavior in several investigated species [79,80].

Prolactin may play a further role in the regulation of clutch size in species producing clutches of more than two eggs [81]. Cessation of egg laying and onset of incubation is linked with an increase in plasma prolactin levels in birds with clutch sizes of more than two eggs [81,82]. Plasma prolactin levels rise with the onset of incubation and the end of laying and therefore, may enhance incubation behavior [81]. In avian species showing hatching asynchrony, prolactin may influence the degree of asynchrony and the clutch size [81]. In the American kestrel (*Falco sparverius*), a species showing pronounced hatching asynchrony, plasma prolactin concentration during egg laying was significantly higher in female birds laying small clutches than in those laying larger clutches [81]. In this species, it is believed that the increasing concentrations of plasma prolactin after the onset of laying leads to a pronounced hatching asynchrony, by the induction of incubating behavior. Embryonic development of early laid eggs may begin before the clutch is completed, leading to pronounced hatching asynchrony, and consequently, to a developmental and competitive hierarchy among siblings, which can have a substantial impact on reproductive success [81].

During incubation, the secretion of LH is depressed and the secretion of prolactin is at its highest. The same endocrine changes occur during the development of reproductive photorefractoriness [51]. In starlings, prolactin plasma levels rise under lengthening daylight periods, with the peak of circulating prolactin temporally linked with the onset of photorefractoriness and the termination of breeding season, which is followed by a postnuptial molt [60,83].

Gonadal hormones

Synthesis and release of gonadal steroidal hormones is controlled predominately by LH and FSH through a negative feedback mechanism by way of the hypothalamus. Besides the steroidal hormones (estrogens, androgens, progesterone), many other factors are produced by the gonads, including inhibin, prostaglandins, and growth factors [46,84].

The production of ovarian steroid hormones depends on the stage of follicular development; the sensitivity of the follicle to gonadotropins; the influence of locally produced factors, including insulin-like growth factors and epidermal growth factor, among others, in synergism with LH and FSH [43]. Growth factors play a role in steroidogenesis, follicular recruitment, and development [43].

Estrogens

Estrogens are produced predominately in the small prehierarchal follicles, but increased production in the four largest hierarchal follicles occurs shortly before ovulation [84].

The plasma concentrations of estrogens are highest 4 to 6 hours before ovulation, coincident with the daily surge of LH and progesterone in the laying female bird [84]. Estrogens have various functions in the reproductive and other organ systems. They control the calcium metabolism necessary for egg shell formation. Estrogens induce their own receptors in the oviduct and progesterone receptors in the ovary and oviduct [84]. Moreover, estrogens induce the synthesis of ovalbumin and other proteins in the oviduct, and vitellogenin and transport proteins in the liver, including those for estrogens, testosterone, cortisol, and thyroxin [84].

Androgens

The exact function and underlying mechanism of androgens in the female ovulation process is not well understood, but testosterone is essential for ovulation [84]. In male birds, androgens control testicular development and spermatogenesis, the development of secondary sexual characteristics, and song system development, and influence territorial and mating behavior.

Progesterone

Progesterone is secreted by the large follicles and is stimulated by the preovulatory surge in LH and induction of ovulation [4,13]. Progesterone receptors are located in the hypothalamus, pituitary gland, oviduct, and preovulatory follicles [13]. Progesterone inhibits the expression of estrogen receptors and hence, has an antagonistic effect on estrogen, particularly in the oviduct [85]. In female budgerigars, treatment with progesterone induced precocious development of tubular glands in the magnum region of the oviduct [75]. Administration of exogenous progesterone causes a preovulatory LH surge, premature ovulation, and induction of premature molt [13].

Inhibin

Inhibin is synthesized in the granulosa cells of the largest three to four ovarian follicles of the female bird and in the testis of the male bird [46,86]. Secretion of inhibin is stimulated by gonadotropins [46]. It is assumed that inhibin, in concert with gonadal steroids, has a negative feedback on gonadotropin release, particularly FSH [46,86,87]. A potential autocrine/paracrine function of inhibin on the steroidogenesis of the ovary is suspected [46].

Hormones of the pineal gland

Melatonin

Until recently, it was accepted that the seasonal changes in melatonin secretion in birds do not regulate reproductive activity, as is the case in mammals [88–90]. Evidence is now strong that melatonin is involved in the regulation of several seasonal processes, including gonadotropin secretion and gonadal activity [91–95]. Melatonin is synthesized and released predominately by the pineal gland, but also by the retina and gut [36,96].

As in mammals, the duration of melatonin release in birds exhibits circadian and seasonal changes [93]. Melatonin is released during the dark phase of the light/dark cycle and the amount of secreted melatonin depends on the length of the dark phase. This control of melatonin release is a very accurate indicator of day length and, by comparing the duration of melatonin release with that of the previous nights, provides information about whether day length is increasing or decreasing. Thus, melatonin is likely involved in encoding the day length and also the time of the year [93]. Three high-affinity melatonin receptors (Mel_{1A}, Mel_{1B}, Mel_{1C}) have been identified in target organs, including neural tissue, immune tissue, intestine, and gonads [89,96]. Because of the expression of melatonin receptors within the ovary and testis, a direct action of melatonin on the gonads is suspected [96–99].

With the recent discovery of GnIH and the detection of melatonin receptors (Mel_{1C}) expressed in GnIH neurons, melatonin is assumed to be the key factor in the control of GnIH expression, as demonstrated in Japanese quail (*Coturnix japonica*) [36]. Animals exposed for 3 weeks to short daylight regimes showed a significant increase in GnIH and a significant decrease in testicular weight, compared with birds exposed to a long daylight regime [36]. When the main sources of endogenous melatonin synthesis were removed by pinealectomy and bilateral enucleation, the expression of GnIH decreased. Consequently, exogenous administration of melatonin resulted in increased expression of GnIH [36]. It was concluded that GnIH expression is photoperiodically controlled by prolonged melatonin release, with increased GnIH expression during short-day periods [36]. The discovery of GnIH and the presence of melatonin receptors on GnIH neurons established a direct link between changes in seasonal daylight and reproductive activity. The action of melatonin on GnIH expression led to an inhibition of LH and subsequently, a suppression of reproductive activity.

Administration of exogenous melatonin has also helped demonstrate the role of melatonin in the control of reproductive activity. A negative effect on reproductive activity in several avian species receiving exogenous melatonin has been documented and a dose- and time-related suppression of LH was found [91,94,95,100,101].

Seasonality of reproduction

For survival and reproductive success, appropriate timing of reproduction is crucial [102]. In seasonal or photoperiodic breeders, the breeding period is determined by seasonal changes in day length. Most species originating from subtropic and temperate zones are seasonal breeding (ie, photostimulated) species. Reproduction in these birds occurs during spring and early summer, when increasing day length coincides with the annual period of maximum food abundance [90,103,104]. Most seasonal breeding species become photostimulated by increased day length, so-called "long-day" breeders. Only a few species are short-day breeders (eg, the emu (*Dromaius novaehollandiae*) and the Emperor penguin (*Aptenodytes forsteri*)) [105].

In so-called "opportunistic breeders," the breeding season is not determined primarily by changes in day length, but by external, unpredictable factors, such as food availability or rain [89,90,106]. In seasonal and opportunistic species, the induction of seasonal reproductive activity is the result of up-regulation of the GnRH system and possible down-regulation of the GnIH system, which results in either transient or permanent increases in gonadal hormone production [89].

Photoperiodic breeders

The molecular mechanisms underlying the photoperiodic response of the gonads remain unknown in all living organisms [102]. Detection of light for reproductive photoperiodic signal transduction in birds is suspected to be extraretinal [107]. In birds, nonpineal, nonretinal deep brain photoreceptors are exclusively responsible for detecting photoperiodic changes, leading to photoperiodic-dependent changes in gonadal activity, which is in contrast to mammals, where the eyes are the only organ mediating photoperiodic changes [102]. The avian pineal gland generates a diurnal pattern of plasma melatonin levels, which encodes the day length [108]. No evidence exists that birds or nonmammalian vertebrates use daily changes in plasma melatonin levels as the primary signal for control of the reproductive system [103]. The current revised model of avian photoperiodic response includes three interacting components: (1) a biologic clock, (2) a GnRH-gonadotropin and VIP-prolactin neuroendocrine axis, and (3) intrinsic activities or as-yet-undetermined inputs of GnRH-I and VIP neurons that are not directly linked with changes in photoperiod [103]. The rhythmic expression of circadian clock genes in the mediobasal hypothalamus of Japanese quail (*Coturnix japonica*) has been reported, and the mediobasal hypothalamus is believed to be the center of photoperiodism [102]. Another explanation as to how photostimulation influences the reproductive axis is the presence of a direct neural communication between the nonpineal, nonretinal deep brain photoreceptors [109].

Furthermore, it has been proposed that the light-induced conversion of the prohormone thyroxine to the bioactive triiodothyronine under long-day light may be involved in the photoperiodic response of the gonads in Japanese quail (*Coturnix japonica*) [110,111]. The lighting conditions necessary to photostimulate seasonal birds vary widely among species. Although most birds breed in spring and summer, some migratory birds are exceptions [103]. During the short-day period, seasonal breeders remain in a photosensitive stage. With increase in day length, they become photostimulated and the reproductive system becomes activated. Photoinduced gonadal growth occurs when light is present for a critical duration of time (12–14 hours) per day in the photosensitive phase. Female birds often respond to a lesser degree to photostimulation during the photosensitive state, and environmental cues such as sufficient food supply, population density, availability of nest sites, presence of a mate, temperature, and humidity all act as cues to reach full reproductive activity [112].

Opportunistic (nonphotoperiodic) breeders

Nonphotic cues, such as rain or food availability, act as key factors for the initiation of breeding in the opportunistic breeder [90]. The neuroendocrine mechanisms by which nonphotic factors influence the reproductive system are poorly understood [113]. In certain ecosystems such as deserts, optimal environmental conditions for breeding may only occur for a short period of the year and therefore, reproductive development is initiated before the onset of optimal environmental conditions to maximize the reproductive process [113]. Although it is hypothesized that gonadal cycles are stimulated primarily by nonphotoperiodic cues, photoperiod-mediated changes in gonadotropin secretion and gonadal activity have been reported in opportunistic breeding species [104,113]. Seasonal gonadal regression, secondary to relative photorefractoriness, offers the possibility of delaying reproduction until midsummer and to continue breeding long after the photoperiod has begun to decline [113]. The underlying mechanisms for the rapid increase in gonadal activity due to environmental cues, such as rain in desert species, are unknown [113]. A role of GnIH in a rapid activation process is suspected [113]. Lesser numbers of GnIH perikarya were found in male rufus-winged sparrows (*Aimophila carpalis*) 20 days after the beginning of an irregular occurring summer monsoon season, compared with 7 days before the monsoon [113]. GnRH-containing perikarya numbers were similar, whereas plasma LH concentrations were higher 20 days after the beginning of the seasonal rainfall [104]. Based on these findings, it was hypothesized that in this opportunistic breeding species, photostimulation in the spring leads to increased GnRH release and, consequently, to gonadotropin release by the pituitary gland, but GnIH-mediated mechanism limits LH release. The occurrence of key environmental cues, such the monsoon season, decreases GnIH-mediated inhibition, and therefore, plasma LH increases and complete reproductive activity is achieved [113]. In contrast to this hypothesis, the injection of GnIH did not have any influence on plasma LH concentrations in opposite to the injection of GnRH in this species [104]. Hence, it was concluded that GnIH might not play a role in the acute mechanism, but might play a role in the seasonal control of LH through inhibitory effects on the GnRH system [104].

Medical intervention in reproduction

The most common form of reproductive abnormality seen by avian veterinarians is excessive or abnormal ovulation. Many species of pet birds, including the cockatiel (*Nymphicus hollandicus*), lovebird (*Agapornis* spp), and zebra finch (*Taeniopygia guttata*) are prone to excessive ovulation, and ovariectomy is not a currently viable surgical procedure because of the anatomy and vascular supply of the avian ovary. Although oviductal removal or hysterectomy is reported in the literature as an effective means of inhibiting ovulation, no long-term follow-up studies document effective cessation of ovulation or the rate of abnormalities related to retention of the ovary (eg, ovarian cysts, internal laying) [114,115]. Species differences in response to oviduct removal (eg, Anseriformes versus Psittaciformes) likely also occur but, again, are poorly documented. Unlike in the commercial production of gallinaceous birds, the focus in pet birds is usually on decreasing fertility or the production of eggs.

Progesterone analogs

The first agents used for the chemically mediated cessation of ovulation in pet birds were analogs of progesterone. The prolonged release product medroxyprogesterone (Depo-Provera; Pfizer Inc.) was used effectively by many practitioners in the 1980s and early 1990s but has received strong cautions or recommendations against its use in female birds [1,8,116]. Reported dosages range widely (5–50 mg/kg) and higher doses may be a contributing factor to some of the reported side effects, such as abnormal weight gain, hepatic lipidosis, thromboembolism, and oviductal dysplasia [7]. The timing of the use of progestins in the ovulation cycle may also be important in reducing side effects but this remains unstudied. Levonorgestrel is a later generation synthetic progestin that has been applied extensively in human contraception. Only one controlled study of progestin use in birds has been performed, in which the effects of medroxyprogesterone and levonorgestrel were evaluated in Japanese quail (*Coturnix japonica*) [117]. Each group of ovulating quail received 40 mg/kg of one of the progestins by intramuscular injection, and was followed for 70 days. The levonorgestrel group ceased laying 2 days after the injection and remained anovulatory for 67 ± 4.7 days. The anovulatory periods for the medroxyprogesterone group were much more variable and of shorter duration [117].

Luteinizing hormone analogs

Human chorionic gonadotropin (HCG) (eg, Chorulon; Intervet Inc.) has a primarily LH agonist action when injected into mammalian and avian patients. Supraphysiologic doses have been used (range 250–1000 IU/kg) that lead to down-regulation of GnRH and pituitary LH gonadotrophs. The nonpulsatile nature of this LH effect also leads to markedly increased progesterone levels that likely ablate the small progesterone spikes required to stimulate preovulatory LH release [1]. The timing of the LH-like surge created by HCG administration is important. Ovulation can be prevented if HCG is administered after the start of seasonal hormonal behavior but before estrogen levels peak (and follicular maturation occurs). If administered during the period of follicular maturation, then ovulation is likely to occur; however, a follow-up dose on day 3 will frequently suppress ovulation. Various dosage schedules have been advocated, ranging from single, large aliquots to alternate-day programs [1,118].

GnRH analogs

Leuprolide acetate (eg, Lupron Depot; TAP Pharmaceutical Products Inc.) is a synthetic superagonist of mammalian GnRH. It has an effective specificity and affinity approximately 50 times greater than native GnRH in the rat [119]. The 1-month depot product is based on a proprietary, microsphere technology that is designed to release the drug proportionally over a 1-month period from a deep intramuscular injection site in humans. The 1-month product has been used most frequently in avian medicine. The steady, nonpulsatile release of leuprolide acetate mimics GnRH and is thought to down-regulate receptors in the pituitary, preventing the release of LH and FSH. Clinical antigonadotropic doses have been reported in the literature for psittacine birds [120,121]. The only controlled study of the use of leuprolide to prevent egg laying in psittacine birds demonstrated the high doses required to achieve this effect in cockatiels [122]. Other studies in racing pigeons (*Columba livia domestica*) and Hispaniolan Amazon parrots (*Amazona ventralis*) showed no or only a weak and short term response to treatment with leuprolide acetate [123,124]. Avian leuprolide acetate doses are higher compared to the doses used for the treatment of precocious puberty in humans or for the chemical castration of men with advanced prostate cancer [125]. The higher requirement leuprolide acetate in birds and the often poor or inconsistent response are likely attributable to the unique structure of avian GnRH receptors [11,29].

Clinical responses to leuprolide acetate, and new information concerning the structure of avian GnRH receptors, suggest that a targeted cGnRH-I agonist would likely be more effective in birds. Currently, no known avian GnRH agonists exist, but research in the chemical design of such a compound is possible and would be rewarding for this application.

Immunocontraception

Although still in its infancy, immunocontraception for pet birds shows future promise. Immunocontraception may have merit as a noninvasive approach for some pet parrots, where breeding is not desired and the deleterious effects of behaviors associated with seasonal hormonal cycling are unacceptable to owners.

In mammals, different approaches are used to develop a contraceptive vaccine. Investigated molecules are targeting either gamete production (GnRH, FSH), gamete function (sperm or zona pellucida antigens), or gamete outcome (HCG) [126]. So far, only GnRH vaccines and anti–zona pellucida vaccines show promising efficacy in mammals.

A vaccine targeting GnRH raises antibodies that bind with the peptide after release from the hypothalamus, preventing passage into the anterior pituitary and stimulation of gonadotropin release. However, the development of a GnRH vaccine for immunocontraception is problematic: because GnRH itself is not immunogenic [126,127]. In order to provoke an immunologic response and the production of antibodies, GnRH has to be conjugated with an antigenetic determinant or carrier to mobilize T-helper cells [126,127].

Long-term contraception is possible and GnRH vaccines have been used successfully in humans and mammals [126–137]. A commercial GnRH vaccine (Improvac; CSL Animal Health) is available in some countries for use in mares.

In chicken, immunization with cGnRH-I or chicken riboflavin carrier protein failed to suppress reproductive activity [138]. The failure was attributed to the vaccination protocol. Future research is necessary to develop a cGnRH-I vaccine with the potential for long-term suppression of the reproductive system in avian species.

Gonadotropin-inhibiting hormone

The application of a slow-release format of GnIH suggests a promising, targeted method of blocking gonadotropin release and thus preventing ovulation in birds. Side effects would be minimal and comparable to the use of an effective, slow-release GnRH agonist. Work in the chicken is proceeding, but no trials in other avian species have yet been performed.

Cholesterol inhibitors

20.25 diazacholesterol

20.25 diazacholesterol (DiazaCon) was investigated originally as a cholesterol-lowering agent in humans [139]. It was further considered as a contraceptive agent in several avian species including pigeons (*Columba livia domestica*), red-winged blackbirds (*Agelaius phoeniceus,*) common grackles (*Quiscalus quiscula*), house sparrows (*Passer domesticus*), and the Japanese quail (*Coturnix japonica*) [140–145]. The early research revealed partially conflicting results regarding the efficiency and side effects. Until 1993, it was registered as an avian pesticide for use in feral pigeons [146]. Lately the potential of Diaza-Con was rediscovered and new research was performed in several avian species, including Japanese quail (*Coturnix japonica,*) mallards (*Anas platyrhynchos,*) American crows (*Corvus brachyrhynchos*), ring-necked doves (*Streptopelia capicola*), and monk parakeets (*Myiopsitta monachus*) [138,146].

DiazaCon is a potent cholesterol synthesis inhibitor, and it acts in several possible ways [146–148]. Cholesterol is the base material for gonadal sex steroid synthesis, and a reduction in the plasma testosterone and progesterone levels, and, consequently, decreased fertility, have been reported after administration of DiazaCon [138,146]. The half-life of DiazaCon in pigeons is 28 days and 50% of orally administered DiazaCon is excreted by feces within 24 hours [149]. DiazaCon is stored in the liver and cleared slowly over time [146].

In Japanese quail (*Coturnix japonica*), oral administration of DiazaCon significantly reduced plasma testosterone levels in male and progesterone levels in female animals, whereas plasma corticosterone levels were not affected. These changes lasted for at least 3 months [138]. Egg production was reduced by 85% and hatchability by 100% in treated female quail [138]. In monk parakeets (*Myiopsitta monachus*), an oral dose of 50 mg/kg every 24 hours for 5 to 7 days resulted in a significant decrease of plasma cholesterol levels for a period of greater than or equal to 3 months [146]. Egg production was reduced by 59% and hatchability by 100% over a 2-month period [146].

Partially severe side effects and mortality were reported in several avian species, because intestinal absorption differs among species [138,146]. Cholesterol is an integral part of the cell membrane and inhibition of the cholesterol synthesis by DiazaCon could have cytotoxic effects. Therefore, further investigation and dose response studies are necessary.

The application of DiazaCon as a contraceptive agent may only be useful in seasonal reproductive species; in these, it has the potential to suppress reproduction for one season after an initial treatment of several days' duration. In nonseasonal breeding species, application is questionable because of the significant cholesterol-lowering effect, which limits the length of treatment because of the increased chance of side effects with prolonged application [146].

Acknowledgments

The authors thank Gregory Bédécarrats for his helpful comments on this article.

References

[1] Pollock CG, Orosz SE. Avian reproductive anatomy, physiology and endocrinology. Vet Clin North Am Exot Anim Pract 2002;5(3):441–74.
[2] Crosta L, Gerlach H, Burkle M, et al. Physiology, diagnosis, and diseases of the avian reproductive tract. Vet Clin North Am Exot Anim Pract 2003;6(1):57–83.
[3] Hudelson K. A review of the mechanisms of avian reproduction and their clinical application. Sem Avian Exotic Pet Med 1996;5(4):189–98.
[4] Ottinger MA, Bakst MR. Endocrinology of the avian reproductive system. J Avian Med Surg 1995;9(4):242–50.
[5] Paster M. Avian reproductive endocrinology. Vet Clin North Am Small Anim Pract 1991; 21(6):1343–59.
[6] Millam JR, et al. Reproductive physiology. In: Altman RB, Clubb SL, Dorrestein GM, editors. Avian medicine and surgery. Philadelphia: WB Saunders; 1997. p. 12–26.
[7] Joyner KL. Theriogenology. In: Ritchie BW, Harrison GJ, Harrison LR, editors. Avian medicine: principles and application. Lake Worth (FL): Wingers; 1994. p. 748–804.
[8] Bowles HL. Evaluating and treating the reproductive system. In: Harrison GJ, Lightfoot TL, editors. Clinical avian medicine, vol. 2Palm Beach: Spix Publishing; 2006. p. 519–40.
[9] Follett BK. Birds. In: Lamming GE, editor. Marshall's physiology of reproduction: reproductive cycles of vertebrates. New York: Churchill Livingstone; 1984. p. 284–350.
[10] Tsutsui K, Bentley GE, Ubuka T, et al. The general and comparative biology of gonadotropin-inhibitory hormone (GnIH). Gen Comp Endocrinol 2007;153(1-3):365–70.
[11] Bédécarrats GY, Shimizu M, Guemene D. Gonadotropin releasing hormone and their receptors in avian species. Journal of Poultry Science 2006;43(3):199–214.
[12] Dunn IC, Millam JR. Gonadotropin releasing hormone: forms and functions in birds. Poultry and Avian Biology Reviews 1998;9(2):61–85.
[13] Scanes CG. Introduction to endocrinology: pituitary gland. In: Whittow CG, editor. Sturkie's avian physiology. 5th edition. New York: Academic Press; 2000. p. 437–60.
[14] Dunn IC, Lewis PD, Wilson PW, et al. Acceleration of maturation of FSH and LH responses to photostimulation in prepubertal domestic hens by n+. Reproduction 2003; 126(2):217–25.
[15] Sharp PJ, Ciccone N. The gonadotropin releasing hormone neurone: key to avian reproductive function. In: Dawson A, Sharp PJ, editors. Functional avian endocrinology. New Dehli: Narosa Publishing House; 2005. p. 59–72.
[16] King JA, Millar RP. Structure of chicken hypothalamic luteinizing hormone-releasing hormone. II. Isolation and characterization. J Biol Chem 1982;257(18):10729–32.
[17] Miyamoto K, Hasegawa Y, Nomura M, et al. Identification of the second gonadotropin-releasing hormone in chicken hypothalamus: evidence that gonadotropin secretion is probably controlled by two distinct gonadotropin-releasing hormones in avian species. Proc Natl Acad Sci USA 1984;81(12):3874–8.

[18] Bentley GE, Moore IT, Sower SA, et al. Evidence for a novel gonadotropin-releasing hormone in hypothalamic and forebrain areas in songbirds. Brain Behav Evol 2004;63(1): 34–46.

[19] Teruyama R, Beck MM. Changes in immunoreactivity to anti-cGnRH-I and -II are associated with photostimulated sexual status in male quail. Cell Tissue Res 2000;300(3): 413–26.

[20] Millam JR, Craig-Veit CB, Adams TE, et al. Avian gonadotropin-releasing hormones I and II in brain and other tissues in turkey hens. Comp Biochem Physiol A 1989;94(4):771–6.

[21] Sharp PJ, Talbot RT, Main GM, et al. Physiological roles of chicken LHRH-I and -II in the control of gonadotrophin release in the domestic chicken. J Endocrinol 1990;124(2):291–9.

[22] Lal P, Sharp PJ, Dunn IC, et al. Absence of an effect of naloxone, an opioid antagonist, on luteinizing hormone release in vivo and luteinizing hormone-releasing hormone I release in vitro in intact, castrated, and food restricted cockerels. Gen Comp Endocrinol 1990;77(2): 239–45.

[23] Mikami S, Yamada S, Hasegawa Y, et al. Localization of avian LHRH-immunoreactive neurons in the hypothalamus of the domestic fowl, Gallus domesticus, and the Japanese quail, Coturnix coturnix. Cell Tissue Res 1988;251(1):51–8.

[24] Clerens S, D'Hondt E, Berghman LR, et al. Identification of cGnRH-II in the median eminence of Japanese quail (Coturnix coturnix japonica). Gen Comp Endocrinol 2003;131(1): 48–56.

[25] van Gils J, Absil P, Grauwels L, et al. Distribution of luteinizing hormone-releasing hormones I and II (LHRH-I and -II) in the quail and chicken brain as demonstrated with antibodies directed against synthetic peptides. J Comp Neurol 1993;334(2):304–23.

[26] Wilson SC, Chairil RA, Cunningham FJ, et al. Changes in the hypothalamic contents of LHRH-I and -II and in pituitary responsiveness to synthetic chicken LHRH-I and -II during the progesterone-induced surge of LH in the laying hen. J Endocrinol 1990;127(3):487–96.

[27] Rozenboim I, Silsby JL, Tabibzadeh C, et al. Hypothalamic and posterior pituitary content of vasoactive intestinal peptide and gonadotropin-releasing hormones I and II in the turkey hen. Biol Reprod 1993;49(3):622–6.

[28] Maney DL, Richardson RD, Wingfield JC. Central administration of chicken gonadotropin-releasing hormone-II enhances courtship behavior in a female sparrow. Horm Behav 1997;32(1):11–8.

[29] Shimizu M, Bedecarrats GY. Identification of a novel pituitary-specific chicken gonadotropin-releasing hormone receptor and its splice variants. Biol Reprod 2006;75(5):800–8.

[30] Barran PE, Roeske RW, Pawson AJ, et al. Evolution of constrained gonadotropin-releasing hormone ligand conformation and receptor selectivity. J Biol Chem 2005;280(46): 38569–75.

[31] Tsutsui K, Saigoh E, Ukena K, et al. A novel avian hypothalamic peptide inhibiting gonadotropin release. Biochem Biophys Res Commun 2000;275(2):661–7.

[32] Ubuka T, Kim S, Huang Y, et al. Gonadotropin-inhibitory hormone neurons interact directly with gonadotropin-releasing hormone-I and -II neurons in European Starling brain. Endocrinol in press.

[33] Bentley GE, Perfito N, Ukena K, et al. Gonadotropin-inhibitory peptide in song sparrows (Melospiza melodia) in different reproductive conditions, and in house sparrows (Passer domesticus) relative to chicken-gonadotropin-releasing hormone. J Neuroendocrinol 2003;15(8):794–802.

[34] Yin H, Ukena K, Ubuka T, et al. A novel G protein-coupled receptor for gonadotropin-inhibitory hormone in the Japanese quail (Coturnix japonica): identification, expression and binding activity. J Endocrinol 2005;184(1):257–66.

[35] Bentley GE, Jensen JP, Kaur GJ, et al. Rapid inhibition of female sexual behavior by gonadotropin-inhibitory hormone (GnIH). Horm Behav 2006;49(4):550–5.

[36] Ubuka T, Bentley GE, Ukena K, et al. Melatonin induces the expression of gonadotropin-inhibitory hormone in the avian brain. Proc Natl Acad Sci USA 2005;102(8):3052–7.

[37] Ubuka T, Ukena K, Sharp PJ, et al. Gonadotropin-inhibitory hormone inhibits gonadal development and maintenance by decreasing gonadotropin synthesis and release in male quail. Endocrinology 2006;147(3):1187–94.

[38] Osugi T, Ukena K, Bentley GE, et al. Gonadotropin-inhibitory hormone in Gambel's white-crowned sparrow (Zonotrichia leucophrys gambelii): cDNA identification, transcript localization and functional effects in laboratory and field experiments. J Endocrinol 2004;182(1):33–42.

[39] Tachibana T, Sato M, Takahashi H, et al. Gonadotropin-inhibiting hormone stimulates feeding behavior in chicks. Brain Res 2005;1050(1–2):94–100.

[40] Proudman JA, Vandesande F, Berghman LR. Immunohistochemical evidence that follicle-stimulating hormone and luteinizing hormone reside in separate cells in the chicken pituitary. Biol Reprod 1999;60(6):1324–8.

[41] Puebla-Osorio N, Proudman JA, Compton AE, et al. FSH- and LH-cells originate as separate cell populations and at different embryonic stages in the chicken embryo. Gen Comp Endocrinol 2002;127(3):242–8.

[42] Bédécarrats GY, Kaiser UB. Differential regulation of gonadotropin subunit gene promoter activity by pulsatile gonadotropin-releasing hormone (GnRH) in perifused L beta T2 cells: role of GnRH receptor concentration. Endocrinology 2003;144(5):1802–11.

[43] Decuypere E, Bruggeman O, Safi M. Endocrine physiology of reproduction in the female chicken: old wine in new bottles. Poultry Avian Biol Rev 2002;13(3):145–53.

[44] Kirby JD, Vizcarra JA, Berghman LR, et al. Regulation of FSH secretion: GnRH independent? In: Dawson A, Sharp PJ, editors. Functional avian endocrinology. New Dehli: Narosa Publishing House; 2005. p. 83–96.

[45] Vanmontfort D, Berghman LR, Rombauts L, et al. Developmental changes in immunoreactive inhibin and FSH in plasma of chickens from hatch to sexual maturity. Br Poult Sci 1995;36(5):779–90.

[46] Johnson PA. Avian inhibin. Poultry Avian Biol Rev 1997;8(2):95–106.

[47] Padmanabhan V, Battaglia D, Brown MB, et al. Neuroendocrine control of follicle-stimulating hormone (FSH) secretion: II. Is follistatin-induced suppression of FSH secretion mediated via changes in activin availability and does it involve changes in gonadotropin-releasing hormone secretion? Biol Reprod 2002;66(5):1395–402.

[48] McCann SM, Karanth S, Mastronardi CA, et al. Control of gonadotropin secretion by follicle-stimulating hormone-releasing factor, luteinizing hormone-releasing hormone, and leptin. Arch Med Res 2001;32(6):476–85.

[49] Vizcarra JA, Kreider DL, Kirby JD. Episodic gonadotropin secretion in the mature fowl: serial blood sampling from unrestrained male broiler breeders (Gallus domesticus). Biol Reprod 2004;70(6):1798–805.

[50] Perera AD, Follett BK. Photoperiodic induction in vitro: the dynamics of gonadotropin-releasing hormone release from hypothalamic explants of the Japanese quail. Endocrinology 1992;131(6):2898–908.

[51] Sharp PJ, Dawson A, Lea RW. Control of luteinizing hormone and prolactin secretion in birds. Comp Biochem Physiol C Pharmacol Toxicol Endocrinol 1998;119(3):275–82.

[52] Dunn IC, Beattie KK, Maney D, et al. Regulation of chicken gonadotropin-releasing hormone-I mRNA in incubating, nest-deprived and laying bantam hens. Neuroendocrinology 1996;63(6):504–13.

[53] Burke WH, Papkoff H. Purification of turkey prolactin and the development of a homologous radioimmunoassay for its measurement. Gen Comp Endocrinol 1980; 40(3):297–307.

[54] Zadworny D, Kansaku N, Bédécarrats G, et al. Prolactin and its receptors in galliformes. Poultry Avian Biol Rev 2002;13(3):223–8.

[55] El Halawani ME, Silsby JL, Rozenboim I, et al. Increased egg production by active immunization against vasoactive intestinal peptide in the turkey (Meleagris gallopavo). Biol Reprod 1995;52(1):179–83.

[56] Kulick RS, Chaiseha Y, Kang SW, et al. The relative importance of vasoactive intestinal peptide and peptide histidine isoleucine as physiological regulators of prolactin in the domestic turkey. Gen Comp Endocrinol 2005;142(3):267–73.

[57] Youngren OM, Pitts GR, Phillips RE, et al. The stimulatory and inhibitory effects of dopamine on prolactin secretion in the turkey. Gen Comp Endocrinol 1995;98(1):111–7.

[58] El Halawani ME, Youngren OM, Rozenboim I, et al. Serotonergic stimulation of prolactin secretion is inhibited by vasoactive intestinal peptide immunoneutralization in the turkey. Gen Comp Endocrinol 1995;99(1):69–74.

[59] Youngren OM, Silsby JL, Phillips RE, et al. Dynorphin modulates prolactin secretion in the turkey. Gen Comp Endocrinol 1993;91(2):224–31.

[60] Goldsmith AR, Nicholls TJ. Prolactin is associated with the development of photorefractoriness in intact, castrated, and testosterone-implanted starlings. Gen Comp Endocrinol 1984;54(2):247–55.

[61] Buntin JD. Neural substrates for prolactin-induced changes in behavior and neuroendocrine function. Poult Sci Rev 1992;4(4):275–87.

[62] Buntin JD, Advis JP, Ottinger MA, et al. An analysis of physiological mechanisms underlying the antigonadotropic action of intracranial prolactin in ring doves. Gen Comp Endocrinol 1999;114(1):97–107.

[63] Reddy IJ, David CG, Raju SS. Effect of suppression of plasma prolactin on luteinizing hormone concentration, intersequence pause days and egg production in domestic hen. Domest Anim Endocrinol 2007;33(2):167-75.

[64] Camper PM, Burke WH. The effect of prolactin on reproductive function in female Japanese quail (Coturnix coturnix japonica). Poult Sci 1977;56(4):1130–4.

[65] Sharp PJ, Macnamee MC, Sterling RJ, et al. Relationships between prolactin, LH and broody behaviour in bantam hens. J Endocrinol 1988;118(2):279–86.

[66] El Halawani ME, Silsby JL, Youngren OM, et al. Exogenous prolactin delays photoinduced sexual maturity and suppresses ovariectomy-induced luteinizing hormone secretion in the turkey (Meleagris gallopavo). Biol Reprod 1991;44(3):420–4.

[67] Buntin JD, Lea RW, Figge GR. Reductions in plasma LH concentration and testicular weight in ring doves following intracranial injection of prolactin or growth hormone. J Endocrinol 1988;118(1):33–40.

[68] Lea RW, Richard-Yris MA, Sharp PJ. The effect of ovariectomy on concentrations of plasma prolactin and LH and parental behavior in the domestic fowl. Gen Comp Endocrinol 1996;101(1):115–21.

[69] Sharp PJ, Blache D. A neuroendocrine model for prolactin as the key mediator of seasonal breeding in birds under long- and short-day photoperiods. Can J Physiol Pharmacol 2003; 81(4):350–8.

[70] El Halawani ME, Rozenboim I. Ontogeny and control of incubation behavior in turkeys. Poult Sci 1993;72(5):906–11.

[71] Book CM, Millam JR, Guinan MJ, et al. Brood patch innervation and its role in the onset of incubation in the turkey hen. Physiol Behav 1991;50(2):281–5.

[72] Massaro M, Setiawan AN, Davis LS. Effects of artificial eggs on prolactin secretion, steroid levels, brood patch development, incubation onset and clutch size in the yellow-eyed penguin (Megadyptes antipodes). Gen Comp Endocrinol 2007;151(2):220–9.

[73] Hall MR, Goldsmith AR. Factors affecting prolactin secretion during breeding and incubation in the domestic duck (Anas platyrhynchos). Gen Comp Endocrinol 1983;49(2):270–6.

[74] El Halawani ME, Silsby JL, Behnke EJ, et al. Hormonal induction of incubation behavior in ovariectomized female turkeys (Meleagris gallopavo). Biol Reprod 1986;35(1):59–67.

[75] Hutchison RE. Effects of ovarian steroids and prolactin on the sequential development of nesting behaviour in female budgerigars. J Endocrinol 1975;67(1):29–39.

[76] Lea RW, Vowles DM, Dick HR. Factors affecting prolactin secretion during the breeding cycle of the ring dove (Streptopelia risoria) and its possible role in incubation. J Endocrinol 1986;110(3):447–58.

[77] Lehrman DS, Brody PN. Effect of prolactin on established incubation behavior in the ring dove. J Comp Physiol Psychol 1964;57(2):161–5.

[78] Janik DS, Buntin JD. Behavorial and physiological effects of prolactin in incubating ring doves. J Endocrinol 1985;105(2):201–9.

[79] Pedersen HC. Effects of exogenous prolactin on parental behaviour in free-living female willow ptarmigan Lagopus l. lagpusi. Anim Behav 1989;38(6):926–34.

[80] Moore CL. Experiential and hormonal conditions affect squab-egg choice in ring doves (Streptopelia risoria). J Comp Physiol Psychol 1976;90(6):583–9.

[81] Sockman KW, Schwabl H, Sharp PJ. The role of prolactin in the regulation of clutch size and onset of incubation behavior in the American kestrel. Horm Behav 2000; 38(3):168–76.

[82] Lea RW, Dods AS, Sharp PJ, et al. The possible role of prolactin in the regulation of nesting behaviour and the secretion of luteinizing hormone in broody bantams. J Endocrinol 1981; 91(1):89–97.

[83] Dawson A, Sharp PJ. The role of prolactin in the development of reproductive photorefractoriness and postnuptial molt in the European starling (Sturnus vulgaris). Endocrinology 1998;139(2):485–90.

[84] Johnson AL. Reproduction in the female. In: Whittow CG, editor. Sturkie's avian physiology. 5th edition. New York: Academic Press; 2000. p. 569–96.

[85] Dougherty DC, Sanders MM. Estrogen action: revitalization of the chick oviduct model. Trends Endocrinol Metab 2005;16(9):414–9.

[86] Johnson PA, Brooks C, Wang SY, et al. Plasma concentrations of immunoreactive inhibin and gonadotropins following removal of ovarian follicles in the domestic hen. Biol Reprod 1993;49(5):1026–31.

[87] Johnson PA, Wang SY. Characterization and quantitation of mRNA for the inhibin alpha-subunit in the granulosa layer of the domestic hen. Gen Comp Endocrinol 1993;90(1): 43–50.

[88] Wilson FE. Neither retinal nor pineal photoreceptors mediate photoperiodic control of seasonal reproduction in American tree sparrows (Spizzela arborea). J Exp Zool 1991;259(1): 117–27.

[89] Gahr M, Fusani L, Jansen R, et al. Melatonin-dependent song pattern of song-birds: bypassing the gonadal control of sexual behavior. In: Dawson A, Sharp PJ, editors. Functional avian endocrinology. New Dehli: Narosa Publishing House; 2005. p. 203–14.

[90] Dawson A, King VM, Bentley GE, et al. Photoperiodic control of seasonality in birds. J Biol Rhythms 2001;16(4):365–80.

[91] Ohta M, Kadota C, Konishi H. A role of melatonin in the initial stage of photoperiodism in the Japanese quail. Biol Reprod 1989;40(5):935–41.

[92] Bentley GE, Ball GF. Photoperiod-dependent and -independent regulation of melatonin receptors in the forebrain of songbirds. J Neuroendocrinol 2000;12(8):745–52.

[93] Bentley GE. Unraveling the enigma: the role of melatonin in seasonal processes in birds. Microsc Res Tech 2001;53(1):63–71.

[94] Guyomarc'h C, Lumineau S, Vivien-Roels B, et al. Effect of melatonin supplementation on the sexual development in European quail (Coturnix coturnix). Behav Processes 2001; 53(1–2):121–30.

[95] Rozenboim I, Aharony T, Yahav S. The effect of melatonin administration on circulating plasma luteinizing hormone concentration in castrated White Leghorn roosters. Poult Sci 2002;81(9):1354–9.

[96] Pang SF, Pang CS, Poon AMS, et al. An overview of melatonin and melatonin receptors in birds. Poultry Avian Biol Rev 1996;7(4):217–28.

[97] Ayre EA, Pang SF. 2-[125I]iodomelatonin binding sites in the testis and ovary: putative melatonin receptors in the gonads. Biol Signals 1994;3(2):71–84.

[98] Ayre EA, Wang ZP, Brown GM, et al. Localization and characterization of [125I]iodomelatonin binding sites in duck gonads. J Pineal Res 1994;17(1):39–47.

[99] Ayre EA, Yuan H, Pang SF. The identification of 125I-labelled iodomelatonin-binding sites in the testes and ovaries of the chicken (Gallus domesticus). J Endocrinol 1992; 133(1):5–11.

[100] Gupta BB, Haldar-Misra C, Ghosh M, et al. Effect of melatonin on gonads, body weight, and luteinizing hormone (LH) dependent coloration of the Indian finch, Lal munia (Estrilda amandava). Gen Comp Endocrinol 1987;65(3):451–6.

[101] Chakraborty S. A comparative study of annual changes in the pineal gland morphology with reference to the influence of melatonin on testicular activity in tropical birds, Psittacula cyanocephala and Ploceus philippinus. Gen Comp Endocrinol 1993;92(1):71–9.

[102] Yoshimura T. Molecular mechanism of the photoperiodic response of gonads in birds and mammals. Comp Biochem Physiol A Mol Integr Physiol 2006;144(3):345–50.

[103] Sharp PJ. Photoperiodic regulation of seasonal breeding in birds. Ann N Y Acad Sci 2005; 1040:189–99.

[104] Deviche P, Small TW, Sharp PJ, et al. Control of luteinizing hormone and testosterone secretion in a flexibly breeding male passerine, the rufous-winged sparrow, Aimophila carpalis. Gen Comp Endocrinol 2006;149(3):226–35.

[105] Malecki IA, Martin GB, O'Malley PJ, et al. Endocrine and testicular changes in a short-day seasonally breeding bird, the emu (Dromaius novaehollandiae), in southwestern Australia. Anim Reprod Sci 1998;53(1–4):143–55.

[106] Small TW, Sharp PJ, Deviche P. Environmental regulation of the reproductive system in a flexibly breeding Sonoran desert bird, the rufous-winged sparrow, Aimophila carpalis. Horm Behav 2007;51(4):483–95.

[107] Kuenzel WJ. The search for deep encephalic photoreceptors within the avian brain, using gonadal development as a primary indicator. Poult Sci 1993;72(5):959–67.

[108] Kumar V, Follett BK. The circadian nature of melatonin secretion in Japanese quail (Coturnix coturnix japonica). J Pineal Res 1993;14(4):192–200.

[109] Saldanha CJ, Silverman AJ, Silver R. Direct innervation of GnRH neurons by encephalic photoreceptors in birds. J Biol Rhythms 2001;16(1):39–49.

[110] Yoshimura T, Yasuo S, Watanabe M, et al. Light-induced hormone conversion of T4 to T3 regulates photoperiodic response of gonads in birds. Nature 2003;426(6963):178–81.

[111] Yasuo S, Watanabe M, Nakao N, et al. The reciprocal switching of two thyroid hormone-activating and -inactivating enzyme genes is involved in the photoperiodic gonadal response of Japanese quail. Endocrinology 2005;146(6):2551–4.

[112] Bentley GE, Audage NC, Hanspal EK, et al. Photoperiodic response of the hypothalamo-pituitary-gonad axis in male and female canaries, Serinus canaria. J Exp Zoolog A Comp Exp Biol 2003;296(2):143–51.

[113] Deviche P, Small T. Environmental control of reproduction in Sonoran desert Aimophila sparrows. In: Dawson A, Sharp PJ, editors. Functional avian endocrinology. New Dehli: Narosa Publishing House; 2005. p. 153–66.

[114] Echols SM. Surgery of the avian reproductive tract. Sem Avian Exotic Pet Med 2002;11(4): 177–95.

[115] Bowles HL, Odberg E, Harrison GJ, et al. Soft tissue disorders. In: Harrison GJ, Lightfoot TL, editors. Clinical avian medicine, vol. 2. Palm Beach: Spix Publishing; 2006. p. 813–8.

[116] Pollock CG, Carpenter JW, Antinoff N. Hormones and steroids used in birds. In: Carpenter JW, editor. Exotic animal formulary. St Louis: Elsevier Saunders; 2005. p. 213–9.

[117] Tell L, Shukla A, Munson L, et al. A comparison of the effects of slow release, injectable levonorgestrel and depot medroxyprogesterone acetate on egg production in Japanese quail. J Avian Med Surg 1999;13(1):23–31.

[118] Lightfoot TL. Clinical use and preliminary data of chorionic gonadotropin administration in psittacines. In: Proceedings of the Association of Avian Veterinarians. Tampa; 1996. p. 303–6.

[119] Ottinger MA, Wu J, Pelican K. Neuroendocrine regulation of reproduction in birds and clinical applications of GnRH analogues in birds and mammals. Sem Avian Exotic Pet Med 2002;11(2):71–9.

[120] Zantop D. Using leuprolide acetate to manage common avian reproductive problems. In: Proceedings of the Second International Conference on Exotics. Fort Lauderdale; 2000. p. 70.

[121] Bowles HL. Update of management of avian reproductive disease with leuprolide acetate. In: Proceedings of the Association of Avian Veterinarians. Orlando (FL); 2001. p. 7–10.

[122] Millam JR, Finney HL. Leuprolide acetate can reversibly prevent egg laying in cockatiels (Nymphicus hollandicus). Zoo Biol 1994;13:149–55.

[123] De Wit M, Westerhof I, Pefold LM. Effect of leuprolide acetate on avian reproduction. In: Proceedings of the Association of Avian Veterinarians. New Orleans (LA) 2004. p. 73–4.

[124] Klaphake E, Greenacre C, Fecteau K, et al. Hormonal effects of leuprolide in Hispaniolan Amazon Parrots. In: Proceedings of the Association of Avian Veterinarians. New Orleans (LA); 2004. p. 353–5.

[125] Pharmaceuticals T. Lupron Depot 7.5 mg and Lupron Depot-Ped package inserts. Lake Forest (IL). 2006.

[126] Naz RK, Gupta SK, Gupta JC, et al. Recent advances in contraceptive vaccine development: a mini-review. Hum Reprod 2005;20(12):3271–83.

[127] Kutzler M, Wood A. Non-surgical methods of contraception and sterilization. Theriogenology 2006;66(3):514–25.

[128] Talwar GP, Raina K, Gupta JC, et al. A recombinant luteinising-hormone-releasing-hormone immunogen bioeffective in causing prostatic atrophy. Vaccine 2004;22(27–28): 3713–21.

[129] Parkinson RJ, Simms MS, Broome P, et al. A vaccination strategy for the long-term suppression of androgens in advanced prostate cancer. Eur Urol 2004;45(2):171–4 [discussion: 174–5].

[130] Tast A, Love RJ, Clarke IJ, et al. Effects of active and passive gonadotrophin-releasing hormone immunization on recognition and establishment of pregnancy in pigs. Reprod Fertil Dev 2000;12(5–6):277–82.

[131] Levy JK, Miller LA, Cynda Crawford P, et al. GnRH immunocontraception of male cats. Theriogenology 2004;62(6):1116–30.

[132] Robbins SC, Jelinski MD, Stotish RL. Assessment of the immunological and biological efficacy of two different doses of a recombinant GnRH vaccine in domestic male and female cats (Felis catus). J Reprod Immunol 2004;64(1–2):107–19.

[133] Jewgenow K, Dehnhard M, Hildebrandt TB, et al. Contraception for population control in exotic carnivores. Theriogenology 2006;66(6–7):1525–9.

[134] Barber MR, Fayrer-Hosken RA. Possible mechanisms of mammalian immunocontraception. J Reprod Immunol 2000;46(2):103–24.

[135] Miller LA, Johns BE, Killian GJ. Immunocontraception of white-tailed deer with GnRH vaccine. Am J Reprod Immunol 2000;44(5):266–74.

[136] Miller LA, Johns BE, Elias DJ, et al. Comparative efficacy of two immunocontraceptive vaccines. Vaccine 1997;15(17–18):1858–62.

[137] Miller LA, Rhyan JC, Drew M. Contraception of bison by GnRH vaccine: a possible means of decreasing transmission of brucellosis in bison. J Wildl Dis 2004;40(4):725–30.

[138] Yoder CA, Andelt WF, Miller LA, et al. Effectiveness of twenty, twenty-five diazacholesterol, avian gonadotropin-releasing hormone, and chicken riboflavin carrier protein for inhibiting reproduction in Coturnix quail. Poult Sci 2004;83(2):234–44.

[139] Sachs BA, Wolfman L. 20, 25-Diazacholestenol dihydrochloride. Inhibition of cholesterol biosynthesis in hyperlipemic subjects. Arch Intern Med 1965;116:366–72.

[140] Lofts B, Murton RK, Thearle RJ. The effects of 22, 25-diazacholesterol dihydrochloride on the pigeon testis and on reproductive behaviour. J Reprod Fertil 1968;15(1):145–8.

[141] Schortmeyer JL, Bechwith SL. Chemical control of pigeon reproduction. In: Transactions of the 35th North American Wildlife and Natural Resources Conference. Washington, DC; 1970. p. 47–55.

[142] Sturtevant J, Wentworth BC. Effect on acceptability and fecundity to pigeon of coating SC 12937 bait with Zein or Ethocel. J Wildl Manage 1970;34:776–82.

[143] Fringer RC, Granett P. The effects of Ornitrol on wild populations of red-winged blackbirds and grackles. In: Proceedings of the 5th Bird Control Seminar. Bowling Green (OH); 1970. p. 163–76.

[144] Sander CW, Elder WH. Oral chemosterilization of the house sparrow. International Pest Control 1976;18:4–8.

[145] Mitchell CJ, Hayes RO, Hughues TBJ. Effects of the chemosterilant Ornitrol on house sparrow reproduction. Am Midl Nat 1979;101:443–6.

[146] Yoder CA, Bynum KS, Miller LA. Development of Diazacon™ as an avian contraceptive. In: Proceedings of the 11th Wildlife Damage Management Conference. Traverse City (MI); 2005. p. 190–201.

[147] Johnston JJ, Goodall MJ, Yoder CA, et al. Desmosterol: a biomarker for the efficient development of 20,25-diazacholesterol as a contraceptive for pest wildlife. J Agric Food Chem 2003;51(1):140–5.

[148] Emmons GT, Rosenblum ER, Peace JN, et al. Effects of 20,25-diazacholesterol on cholesterol synthesis in cultured chick muscle cells: a radiogas chromatographic and mass spectrometric study of the post-squalene sector. Biomed Mass Spectrom 1982;9(7):278–85.

[149] Klimstra PD, Ranney RE, Counsell RE. Hypocholesterolemic agents. VI. A- and B-ring-modified azacholesterols. J Med Chem 1966;9(3):323–6.

ELSEVIER
SAUNDERS

Vet Clin Exot Anim 11 (2008) 107–123

VETERINARY
CLINICS
Exotic Animal Practice

Pancreatic Endocrinopathies in Ferrets

Sue Chen, DVM, DABVP–Avian

*Gulf Coast Avian and Exotics, Gulf Coast Veterinary Specialists, 1111 West Loop South,
Suite 110, Houston, TX 77027, USA*

The domestic ferret (*Mustela putorius furo*) has become an increasingly popular companion animal because of its inquisitive nature and engaging personality. As pet ownership of ferrets has increased over the last 2 decades, the incidence of various endocrinopathies has also increased. Especially common are two types of endocrine neoplasms, pancreatic beta islet cell tumors and adrenocortical neoplasia [1,2]. This article focuses primarily on pancreatic beta islet cell tumors, also known as insulinomas, but also discusses other, less commonly encountered, pancreatic endocrinopathies, such as diabetes mellitus. Information on adrenocortical neoplasia can be found in an associated chapter in this volume of *Veterinary Clinics*.

Pancreatic endocrinopathies appear to occur regionally because most of these tumors occur in North America. A few cases of beta cell tumors have been reported in the Netherlands, Australia, and the United Kingdom, although they are still rare, compared with North America [2–4]. Domestic pet ferrets in the United States are supplied by a small number of breeders, thus limiting their genetic diversity and leading to the hypothesis that the development of insulinomas may have a genetic component [1,2]. The black-footed ferret (*Mustela nigripes*), an endangered and genetically distinct species in the United States, is not plagued by the same type of endocrine neoplasms. In one study investigating the epidemiology of neoplasia in black-footed ferrets, although neoplastic tumors were noted in 55.4% (102 of 184) ferrets at the time of death, none of these ferrets had evidence of beta cell tumors [5].

Another theory about the development of endocrine disease in ferrets focuses on the type of diet offered. Most pet ferrets in the United States are fed a commercial kibble diet, which is in contrast to the whole prey diet that many ferrets are fed in the United Kingdom [6]. The commercial diets are much higher in carbohydrates and may have a negative effect on

E-mail address: drchen@gcvs.com

doi:10.1016/j.cvex.2007.09.001   *vetexotic.theclinics.com* glucose metabolism in ferrets, which are carnivorous. It is thought that the difference in diet, in combination with different husbandry conditions (outdoor versus indoor), may contribute to the propensity of endocrinopathies in ferrets in the United States.

Anatomy and physiology of the pancreas

The pancreas is a light pink-to-tan lobulated organ consisting of two limbs (Fig. 1). The left limb lies within the mesoduodenum, between the greater curvature of the stomach and the spleen. It is bordered by the portal vein and left kidney dorsally and by the transverse colon and jejunoileum ventrally. The right limb is the larger of the two limbs and extends several centimeters dorsomedial along the descending duodenum. It is bordered dorsally by the caudal vena cava, aorta, right kidney, and caudate lobe of the liver. The intestines lie ventral to the right limb. The two limbs are united midline in a region just caudal to the pylorus [7,8].

The ferret's pancreas contains exocrine and endocrine portions and is thought to function similarly to that of other carnivorous mammalian species. The endocrine pancreas comprises only 2% of the total pancreatic

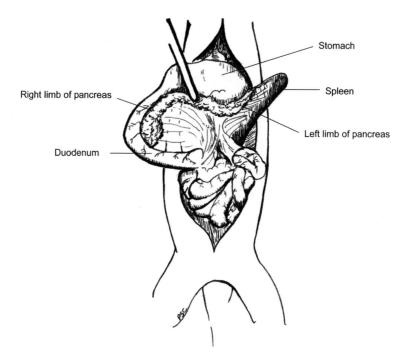

Fig. 1. Ferret abdominal cavity illustrating the pancreas. Stomach is retracted cranially and the dorsal view of the stomach is illustrated.

tissue and consists of at least four types of neuroendocrine cells arranged into groups as islets of Langerhans [9]. Each cell type secretes a single hormone; alpha cells secrete glucagon, beta cells secrete insulin, delta cells secrete somatostatin, and pancreatic polypeptide (PP) cells secrete pancreatic polypeptide [9,10]. It is theorized that these islet cells develop from a common precursor in the primitive gut wall and are a part of a neuroendocrine system made up of amine precursor uptake and decarboxylation cells [11]. Disorders of these cells include abnormal hormone production and secretion; their tumors are often named after the hormone that that particular cell secretes (ie, insulinoma). The acini make up the exocrine portion of the pancreas and secrete digestive juices into the gastrointestinal tract. As with other mammalian species, the presence of capillary connections from the endocrine to the exocrine pancreatic tissues supports the theory that the endocrine pancreas influences the function of the exocrine pancreas [12]. Although rare, exocrine pancreatic adenocarcinomas have also been described [13].

Endocrine pancreatic physiology

The pancreas plays a major role in glucose, lipid, and protein metabolism through the balance of its two major hormones, insulin and glucagon. Insulin, a peptide produced by beta islet cells, is released when levels of glucose, amino acids, and free fatty acids are increased in the blood. In the case of increasing blood glucose concentrations, plasma insulin levels can increase almost 10 fold within minutes of a sudden increase in blood glucose levels. Insulin then causes rapid uptake of glucose into peripheral tissues and promotes the storage of glucose as glycogen in the muscle and liver. Additionally, insulin inhibits hepatic gluconeogenesis and glycogenolysis, and promotes the conversion of excess glucose into fatty acids [10]. The net effect of all these processes is a decrease in blood glucose levels.

Glucagon is secreted by alpha cells in response to decreasing glucose levels and is involved in effects that are exactly opposite to those of insulin, namely, an increase in blood glucose levels. Glucagon increases blood glucose concentrations by stimulating glycogenolysis and gluconeogenesis. In most mammalian species, the insulin feedback mechanism plays a greater role in maintaining a normal blood glucose concentration. However, in instances of excessive glucose use (ie, exercise) or starvation, glucagon does play a valuable role in maintaining normoglycemia [10]. In cases of severe hypoglycemia or stress, other nonpancreatic hormones, such as epinephrine, growth hormone, and cortisol, may be secreted to help return a patient to normal glucose levels [8,10].

Somatostatin, another pancreatic islet hormone, is secreted and produced by delta cells. Somatostatin is released in response to factors related to the ingestion of food, such as increases in glucose, amino acid, and fatty acids levels in the blood stream. This hormone inhibits the secretion of insulin and glucagon and decreases the gastrointestinal motility of the stomach and duodenum [10]. The islets also have a small number of PP cells, which secrete pancreatic polypeptide. The effects of this hormone are poorly understood, but it is thought to stimulate various effects on the gastrointestinal tract, including gastric acid secretion, gastrointestinal motility, and gastric emptying times [10,11].

Endocrine pancreatic disorders

Insulinoma

Pancreatic islet beta cell tumors, more commonly known as insulinomas, have been well recognized and well documented in ferrets over the last 20 years. Numerous retrospective clinical studies document the incidence, clinical disease, and treatment of insulinoma in ferrets [14–17]. In two large retrospective studies, insulinoma was by far the most common neoplasm seen in middle-aged to older ferrets, with a reported incidence of 25% (382 of 1525) and 21.7% (139 or 574) of neoplasms diagnosed [1,14]. Most ferrets begin exhibiting clinical signs around 4 to 6 years of age, although a functional insulinoma has been reported in a ferret as young as 2 weeks old [14]. Both sexes are represented, although reports are conflicting as to whether male ferrets are slightly overrepresented [1,17].

Pathophysiology

Pancreatic β cell tumors produce their effects through the overproduction of insulin. These tumors secrete insulin indiscriminately and are not responsive to inhibitory stimuli such as hypoglycemia and hyperinsulinemia. Additionally, a rapidly increasing glucose level, even in the presence of a low blood glucose concentration, can stimulate excessive insulin release from these tumors, causing a profound rebound hypoglycemia [18]. Although local tumor recurrence is a common feature, metastasis to other organs appears to be low. When it does occur, the regional lymph nodes, liver, and spleen have been the most commonly reported [18–20]. This finding is in contrast to insulinomas found in dogs, which are usually malignant and have a high rate of gross metastasis at time of diagnosis [21].

Clinical signs

Clinical signs include mental dullness, irritability, star-gazing, hind limb weakness, and ataxia. Other common signs noted in ferrets include ptyalism or pawing at the mouth. In these cases, owners may present the ferret with concern that the patient has swallowed a noxious substance or "has something stuck in the mouth." These clinical signs are presumed to be caused by nausea. Alternatively, the ferret may be experiencing numbness or a tingling sensation of the oral cavity, which may be similar to what some people with diabetes experience during an insulin-induced hypoglycemic crisis. Less commonly, severely hypoglycemic ferrets may exhibit generalized seizures, which is the most common clinical finding in dogs with insulinomas [21]. This difference between dogs and ferrets may be due to an inherent difference between species in their tolerance to hypoglycemia or to a difference in husbandry. The ad libitum feeding schedule and low activity lifestyle associated with cage restriction may contribute to the relatively low incidence of generalized seizures in pet ferrets [22]. Clinical signs are often episodic, but the severity and frequency of clinical signs often progress if left untreated [23]. Prolonged episodes of severe hypoglycemia can result in neuronal glucose deprivation and cerebral hypoxia, leading to subsequent lesions in the cerebral cortex [24].

Diagnosis

A presumptive diagnosis of insulinoma is made in ferrets when they demonstrate a fasting blood glucose of less than 60 mg/dL in the presence of neurologic symptoms, and these symptoms cease after a feeding or intravenous administration of glucose (Whipple's triad) [23,25]. Although a fasting blood glucose of less than 60 to 70 mg/dL is suggestive of an insulinoma, other causes of hypoglycemia, such as sepsis, starvation, hepatic disease, and lab artifact, should be ruled out. Immediate evaluation of freshly drawn blood with a handheld glucometer provides a quick relative assessment of the blood glucose status. If a sample is to be sent to a diagnostic laboratory, blood should be collected in a sodium fluoride tube and immediately centrifuged. These measures minimize red cell metabolism because glucose levels will artifactually decrease by approximately 7% per hour if left in contact with red blood cells at room temperature [8]. In patients where an insulinoma is suspected but the blood glucose is within normal limits (80–120 mg/dL), a carefully monitored 3- to 4-hour fast may be required to confirm hypoglycemia.

Plasma or serum obtained during episodes of hypoglycemia can also be submitted for insulin levels at laboratories that have validated the assay for ferrets [26]. Normal insulin concentrations have been reported to be between 4.88 and 34.84 µU/ml (35–250 pmol/L) [8]. However, it is advisable to take into consideration what a particular laboratory's reference values are and what method of assay is used, because different commercial radioimmunoassay kits are not equal [8,27]. Elevated insulin levels (>279 µU/ml) with concurrent hypoglycemia is consistent with hyperinsulinism and supports the diagnosis of an insulinoma [18,24]. However, a normal or low insulin level does not necessarily rule out the presence of an insulinoma if there is erratic production and secretion of insulin [28].

Various insulin-to-glucose ratios, including the amended insulin/glucose ratio, have been used in the past to diagnose the presence of an insulinoma. However, because of their high incidence of false-positives, their use is no longer recommended [8,18]. Although the use of fructosamine and glycosylated hemoglobin (GHb) have not been validated in ferrets yet, studies in people and dogs have demonstrated a direct relationship between serum glucose levels and fructosamine and GHb concentrations [29,30]. Further studies are warranted to determine if these tests can be used to aid in the diagnosis and management of insulinoma cases in ferrets. Provocative tests used in other species have not demonstrated any additional benefit over the simple measurement of glucose and insulin levels and have not been tested in ferrets to date [18].

Other changes in blood work are usually unremarkable and, if present, may be a result of concurrent disease. Findings may include leukocytosis, characterized by a mature neutrophilia and monocytosis. Nonspecific elevations in alanine aminotransferase and aspartate aminotransferase are sometime noted and may reflect the presence of hepatic lipidosis from chronic hypoglycemia [18,21].

Diagnostic imaging, such as radiography and ultrasonography, is usually unrewarding because most insulinomas are only a few millimeters in diameter and may even be microscopic. In rare instances, tumors can be as large as 1 cm in diameter and may represent insulinomas that were medically managed long term without surgical intervention. In these cases, a pancreatic mass may then be noted on ultrasonographic examination.

Histology is required for definitive diagnosis and is acquired through surgical biopsies. Most pancreatic islet cell tumors consist of cords and nests of eosinophilic polyhedral cells on a fine fibrovascular stroma. Although these tumors are usually well circumscribed, some tumors can be infiltrative. Tumors may be described as hyperplasia, adenomas, or carcinomas, and a specific tumor may have a combination of any of these processes. Immunohistochemistry has been used to characterize pancreatic islet cell tumors and associated metastatic masses further. Although immunostaining for peptide hormones such as glucagon, somatostatin, and pancreatic polypeptide has been noted occasionally, most islet cell tumors express strong immunoreactivity for insulin [19,31]. Further studies by Andrews and Myers [31] have demonstrated that neuroendocrine markers chromogranin A and neuron-specific enolase were also effective immunocytochemical markers for ferret islet cell tumors. These markers would be useful in characterizing neuroendocrine tumors of poorly differentiated pancreatic tumors or metastasis in distant organs that may be insulin negative.

Treatment
Surgery. Surgical excision is considered the treatment of choice for greater clinical resolution and longer survival times [18,21,27]. In preparation for surgery, an intravenous catheter should be placed preoperatively to provide maintenance fluids with 5% dextrose pre- and perioperatively to prevent a hypoglycemic crisis [28]. Careful visualization with gentle palpation of the pancreas is performed to locate the pancreatic nodules. Pancreatic nodules can be removed individually or, in the case of multiple nodules,

a partial pancreatectomy can be performed. In one study, ferrets with partial pancreatectomies often had longer survival times than those with nodulectomies [32]. It is presumed that microscopic tumors may be missed by a surgeon when a nodulectomy is performed, versus when a pancreatic limb is removed. A small clinical study in dogs has demonstrated the use of 1% methylene blue administered intravenously to enhance visualization of neoplastic tissue. This dye is preferentially absorbed by hyperfunctional tumor tissue in the endocrine pancreas. Adverse affects can include pseudo-cyanosis from damage and lysis of red blood cells (ie, Heinz bodies) [33]. Use of methylene blue to increase visualization of pancreatic tumors has not been described in ferrets. Intraoperative ultrasound of the pancreas has been also been described in humans and dogs to identify nodules; however, the accuracy depends on operator experience [9,24]. A full abdominal exploratory is recommended to evaluate for areas of potential metastasis and any concurrent conditions such as adrenocortical neoplasia. Biopsies of any suspicious tissues should be collected for histologic evaluation. Postoperative complications such as pancreatitis and hyperglycemia appear to be uncommon in ferrets [24].

Although the ideal goal is for patients to be normoglycemic after surgery, some may remain hypoglycemic and many will have a recurrence of clinical signs several months later because of tumor metastasis. Case studies have demonstrated that as many as 52% (26 out of 50) of ferrets remained hypoglycemic after surgery, and reported disease-free intervals have ranged from 0 to 23.5 months (medians of 234 days, 240 days, and 10.6 months) [17,25,32]. Because of the likely recurrence of signs, owners should be advised that surgery should not be considered curative, but that it may temporarily stop or slow the progression of disease for a longer disease-free interval. In one study, the type of surgery technique had an effect on survival times; nodulectomy combined with partial pancreatectomy had a significantly longer median survival time (668 days), compared with nodulectomy alone (456 days) or medical treatment only (186 days) [32]. Although some patients may need continued medical management of their hypoglycemia after surgery, clinical signs may often be controlled on lower doses of medication. In some cases, ferrets may exhibit an iatrogenic hyperglycemia postoperatively after a partial pancreatectomy. Many of these cases of hyperglycemia are transient and resolve on their own within a few weeks, without treatment or with minimal supportive care [18].

Medical therapy

Symptomatic therapy. Glucocorticoids, such as prednisone and prednisolone, increase the blood glucose level by increasing hepatic gluconeogenesis, decreasing glucose uptake by peripheral tissues, and inhibiting insulin binding to insulin receptors [34]. Doses of 0.25 to 2 mg/kg by mouth every 12 hours have been used [18,35]. Many clinicians start at a low dose and increase the dose incrementally as needed to control clinical symptoms.

Initially, the blood glucose is rechecked in 5 to 7 days and the dose is adjusted as needed to achieve normoglycemia. Although ferrets often are relatively resistant to the immunosuppressive effects of prednisolone, the authors have noted at their clinic that ferrets on long-term glucocorticoid therapy often gain weight in the abdominal region and may have slow or impaired hair growth in any shaved areas.

Diazoxide, a nondiuretic benzothiadiazide, can be added to the treatment regimen when glucocorticoids alone no longer control clinical symptoms. Diazoxide directly inhibits pancreatic insulin secretion by decreasing the intracellular release of ionized calcium, which subsequently prevents the release of insulin from insulin granules. Additionally, diazoxide stimulates the release of epinephrine, which, in turn, promotes hepatic gluconeogenesis and glycogenolysis and decreases cellular uptake of glucose [18,24]. Recommended dosing starts at 5 to 10 mg/kg by mouth every 12 hours, and is gradually increased to a maximum of 30 mg/kg every 12 hours if lower doses do not control signs adequately [35]. Adverse side effects typically include anorexia and vomiting. Additionally, this medication should be used cautiously in patients that have renal disease or congestive heart failure because it can cause sodium and fluid retention [34].

Octreotide is a synthetic, long-acting analog of somatostatin that inhibits the secretion of insulin, glucagon, secretin, gastrin, and motilin [24,34,36]. Limited use of this drug has been reported in the veterinary literature, but it may be useful in some insulinoma patients that are refractory to other types of treatment. Not all insulinomas are responsive to this medication because pancreatic islet cell tumors have varied expression of somatostatin receptors. If an insulinoma does not have somatostatin receptors (as seen in approximately 40% of human cases), the administration of octreotide may exacerbate hypoglycemia because of the suppression of glucagons [36]. The recommended dosage is 1 to 2 µg/kg every 12 to 18 hours subcutaneously [24]. Probably because of the variable presence of somatostatin receptors in each insulinoma, the sporadic use of octreotide in ferrets has produced equivocal results [17,18,24].

Chemotherapy. The aforementioned medications only treat the clinical symptoms and do not have antineoplastic properties. Studies in dogs have shown that streptozocin, an antineoplastic antibiotic, has direct toxic effects on pancreatic beta cells [20,24]. Aggressive saline diuresis is required during drug administration to minimize the development of nephrotoxicosis [34]. Alloxan, another chemotherapeutic, also has a direct toxic effect on pancreatic beta cells. This drug has many associated renal, hepatic, and pulmonary toxicities, and also requires aggressive fluid therapy during administration to prevent renal tubular necrosis [24]. Both these chemotherapeutic drugs are considered investigational in their use in dogs; their use in ferrets has not been evaluated and should be approached with caution because of their many toxic side effects.

Doxorubicin is another antibiotic with antineoplastic effects and may be effective in the treatment of insulinomas. This drug is used widely in veterinary oncology and has been used safely in ferrets as part of chemotherapy protocols for the treatment of lymphoma [20]. Proposed investigational dosing for the treatment of insulinomas is 30 mg/m^2 intravenously every 3 weeks [24,34]. This drug must be administered slowly intravenously and requires precise venipuncture because inadvertent extravasation can result in severe tissue necrosis. Other reported side effects include bone marrow suppression, gastroenteritis, nephrotoxicity, and cardiac toxicity; thus, it is recommended that the cumulative dose be limited to less than 240 mg/m^2 [34].

Diet modification. Equally important in the management of insulinomas is a change in diet. Owners should be instructed to discontinue all treats that are high in simple sugars, including raisins, peanut butter, and any ferret supplements containing corn syrup or other sugar product. The rapid increase of blood glucose from the ingestion of these simple sugars can induce a rebound release of insulin, thus triggering a hypoglycemic episode [37]. Changing to a high-protein, low-carbohydrate diet helps decrease the consumption of simple carbohydrates. It is important for owners to make sure the ferret accepts the new diet because some ferrets can be picky and will go into a hypoglycemic crisis from not eating. Additionally, food should be available at all times. In homes where ferrets are allowed to run free in a ferret-proofed area, owners should be instructed to place food in multiple locations so that it is easily accessible.

Management of a hypoglycemic episode. If an insulinoma is confirmed or suspected, owners should be instructed on measures to minimize clinical signs to provide the ferret a good quality of life. In addition to medical management and diet modification, owners need to know what measures to take during a hypoglycemic episode. Owners should be advised about the clinical signs to look for, such as lethargy or excessive salivation. If clinical signs such as these are noted, owners should provide a feeding to abate the clinical sign. If the owner finds his/her ferret comatose or exhibiting seizures, he/she should drip Karo syrup or a sugar solution on the mucous membranes to provide temporary relief for the hypoglycemia until the ferret can be transported to a veterinary facility for supportive care.

If a ferret is comatose or seizing on presentation to the clinic, the blood glucose level should be assessed quickly for hypoglycemia and an intravenous catheter should be placed immediately for a slow bolus of 50% dextrose (0.25–2 mL) and titrate to effect [18]. Once the seizures have ceased, the patient should be placed on maintenance fluids with 5% dextrose. If a ferret continues to seizure despite an intravenous dextrose bolus, diazepam may be required to stop the seizures.

Pancreatic polypeptidoma

The presence of other neuroendocrine tumors in the pancreas may be underreported because the clinical effects of the beta cell tumors may mask the effects of other tumors in the pancreas. Pancreatic polypeptide-producing tumors are the most common tumor noted in humans with multiple endocrine neoplasia, a clinical syndrome characterized by tumors in the parathyroid gland, anterior pituitary, and pancreatic neuroendocrine islets [11,38]. Clinical signs of pancreatic polypeptidomas are usually secondary to the tumor's mass effect, rather than hormone secretion. However, these tumors can occur concurrently with other functional pancreatic tumors such as insulinomas, gastrinomas, and glucagonomas [38]. A case study evaluating a ferret with multiple endocrine pancreatic tumors where pancreatic polypeptide was the dominant hormone released has been described. This research ferret had basal (216 pg/mL [normal 55.6 pg/mL]) and meal-stimulated (325 pg/mL [normal 80.8 pg/mL]) hypergastrinemia and a presumptive diagnosis of gastrinoma was made. However, the patient did not respond to provocative tests to support this diagnosis. The patient also had elevated levels of pancreatic polypeptide (531 pg/mL [normal <37 pg/mL]) and elevated nonfasting insulin levels (33 μU/ml [normal 12 μU/ml]). On hormone extraction of two of the five pancreatic tumors noted on necropsy, the levels of pancreatic polypeptide were significantly elevated, confirming the diagnosis of this particular type of pancreatic tumor [11].

Diabetes mellitus

Although diabetes mellitus is a widely recognized and studied condition in humans, dogs, and cats, it is an uncommon condition in ferrets. In contrast to insulinomas, diabetes in ferrets is not well documented in the veterinary literature. This syndrome is characterized by the impaired metabolism of carbohydrates, fats, and protein caused by decreased levels of circulating insulin or the development of insulin resistance [10]. Spontaneous diabetes was first described in a black-footed ferret in 1977, and only a few sporadic reports have been noted since then [39]. Hillyer [40] reported treating four middle-aged ferrets with insulin for persistent hyperglycemia. More recently, another case documented diabetes mellitus in a 2-year-old female ferret, where the ferret had been fed a diet solely of sweet cereals for over a year [41]. Most cases of hyperglycemia are usually transient, and are noted as a postsurgical complication after resection of an insulinoma. The paucity of reports may be further decreased because of underreporting, because many practitioners may manage diabetic ferrets as they would a feline diabetic patient. Nevertheless, hyperglycemia is a relatively uncommon endocrinopathy in ferrets.

Pathophysiology

Diabetes mellitus is classified by two different methods. One method is based on the pathogenesis of the disease and uses the classifications, type

1 or type 2. Type 1 patients usually have insulin insufficiency from immune-mediated destruction of either pancreatic beta cells or insulin. In contrast, type 2 diabetics usually are characterized by peripheral insulin resistance, but also may concurrently have altered insulin secretion from beta cell dysfunction [42]. The terms insulin-dependent diabetes mellitus (IDDM) and non–insulin-dependent diabetes mellitus (NIDDM) describe the requirement for exogenous insulin. With IDDM, patients have low insulin concentrations and require insulin for treatment. Patients that have NIDDM are able to produce insulin initially, but the target tissues are insulin resistant. To compensate for the decreased sensitivity to insulin, these patients typically have elevated insulin levels early in the course of the disease. However, with chronic hyperglycemia, the beta cells can become "exhausted" over time and are unable to produce more insulin [10,42]. Although these terms are often used interchangeably, the classification schemes describe different aspects of the disease and are not equal. For example, although most type 1 diabetes mellitus patients are insulin dependent, patients that have type 2 diabetes mellitus can be either insulin or non–insulin dependent and can even change from one to the other through the course of the disease [42].

Because reports of spontaneous diabetes mellitus in ferrets are few, it has not been determined which type seems to afflict this species. In the two ferret cases where histologic evaluation of the pancreas was performed, histologic stains demonstrated an adequate number of beta granules in the pancreatic islets, suggesting that the diabetes was a result of either inadequate release of insulin or a peripheral resistance to insulin [39,41]. Hyperglycemia can also be caused by excessive glucagon secretion from a glucagonoma (alpha cell tumor); however, glucagonomas are rarely reported in people and dogs and currently, no reports have been published about this type of neoplasm in ferrets [9]. Typically, people and dogs with alpha islet cell tumors are hyperglycemic and hypoaminoacidemic, and present with a superficial necrolytic dermatitis [9,43].

Various environmental factors have also been associated with the development of hyperglycemia, including diet, obesity, stress, diabetogenic drugs (ie, steroids), and trauma to the pancreas [42]. Diets high in refined sugar may result in "glucose toxicity," wherein chronic exposure to hyperglycemia impairs beta-cell function and thereby decreases insulin release [41,42]. Increased levels of insulin, corticosteroids, and growth hormone can also result in the down-regulation of insulin receptors, and subsequent hyperglycemia [42]. Hyperglycemia in ferrets is noted most commonly as a postsurgical sequela of insulinoma resection. It is thought that normal pancreatic islet cells may be temporarily suppressed by tumor-derived insulin and a lag time is required for the production of insulin, or that the insulin receptors may be down-regulated from the previously persistent hyperinsulinemia [12,42].

Clinical signs

Ferrets with diabetes may have signs of lethargy, weight loss, polyphagia, polydipsia, and polyuria [39,41,44]. Weakness in the rear limbs, and ataxia, may be noted if a diabetic neuropathy develops [45]. Long-term hyperglycemia can cause structural damage to blood vessels, resulting in a decreased blood supply to multiple tissues and leading to an increased risk for a heart attack, stroke, kidney disease, retinal disease (blindness), and ischemia, with subsequent gangrene of the limbs [10]. Patients that have coexisting disorders such as pancreatitis, infection, or renal disease also have a greater potential for developing ketoacidosis as the body shifts from carbohydrate to fat metabolism. With the development of ketoacidosis, patients become progressively more lethargic, depressed, and tachypneic, and may develop gastrointestinal signs such as vomiting and abdominal pain [45].

Diagnosis

A diagnosis of diabetes is based on appropriate clinical signs, a persistent blood glucose concentration more than 400 mg/dL, and glucosuria [18,45]. Concurrent ketonuria may be present if the patient has become ketoacidotic. In establishing whether or not a ferret is diabetic, physiologic causes of hyperglycemia should be ruled out. Epinephrine released during acute stress can trigger glycolysis to increase blood glucose levels, whereas chronic stress can stimulate an increase in adrenocorticosteroids to prompt an increase in glycolysis and gluconeogenesis [8]. In cases of stress hyperglycemia, these patients usually will not have glucosuria because glucose does not have time to accumulate in the urine with a transient hyperglycemia [45].

A low insulin level in the face of hyperglycemia further supports the diagnosis of diabetes mellitus. However, a normal or elevated insulin level does not rule out diabetes and is suggestive of insulin-resistance or the presence of a glucagonoma. Glucagonomas are rarely reported in any species and no reports in ferrets have been documented. The insulin levels should be evaluated by a diagnostic laboratory that has validated the test for ferrets [27]. In human, canine, and feline patients, fructosamine and GHb concentrations have been used to document persistent hyperglycemia [29,46]. These tests may be beneficial in evaluating if ferrets are persistently or transiently hyperglycemic; however, these tests have not been studied in ferrets and should be validated before their use is recommended. A complete blood count and serum biochemistry panel are recommended to evaluate for any concurrent conditions. Imaging diagnostics such as radiography and ultrasonography do not aid in the diagnosis of diabetes mellitus, but are recommended if any coexisting diseases are suspected.

Histopathologic lesions are similar to those found in other species with diabetes mellitus. In one reported case, the ferret had diffusely and markedly vacuolated Langerhans' islet cells. These cells were positive for insulin on immunoperoxidase staining, thus confirming them as β-cells. The material in the vacuoles was periodic acid–Schiff (PAS) positive and would disappear with amylase digestion, thus confirming the presence of glycogen [41]. Arteriosclerosis and hepatic lipidosis have also been reported in diabetic ferrets and would be consistent with secondary histopathologic lesions seen in people with diabetes [10,39].

Treatment

Therapy is aimed at trying to normalize the blood glucose concentration without the development of hypoglycemia. Because of the low incidence of spontaneous diabetes mellitus in ferrets, few ferret-specific treatment protocols have been described. The current recommendations are based on studies in people and cats; continued advancements in the diagnosis and management of diabetes in other species can, and should, be used in the management of cases in ferrets. Before instituting treatment for diabetes mellitus, veterinarians should take note that if the hyperglycemia is a postoperative complication from insulinoma resection, many of these cases may not require specific therapy and will resolve on their own in a few weeks.

Reported insulin doses used in ferrets include neutral protamine Hagedorn, 0.5 to 1 U per ferret subcutaneously every 12 hours [18]. At the authors' clinic, they have also used Ultralente insulin, starting with 1 U per ferret and gradually increasing the dose until the patient was no longer glucosuric or ketonuric. This ferret was maintained on 3 U twice a day in combination with a low-carbohydrate, high-protein diet, eventually leading to diabetic remission 5 months later. Insulin types and strengths should not be confused because the pharmacokinetics of various formulations can differ greatly. Recently, insulin analogs have been used increasingly in veterinary medicine for their improved pharmacodynamic properties. Glargine, a long-acting synthetic insulin analog, is considered to be a peakless insulin with a long duration of action [46]. Studies in cats have demonstrated a longer duration of action, good-to-moderate glycemic control, and a higher percentage of diabetic remission where the patients no longer requires insulin to maintain normoglycemia [46,47]. Although no published reports of its use in ferrets exist, a long-acting insulin such as glargine may be more suitable, with the feeding strategy most ferrets have. Regardless of type of insulin administered, owners are instructed to check the urine daily for glucosuria and ketonuria with urine dipsticks to confirm hyperglycemia before administering the insulin.

Oral hypoglycemic drugs, such as sulfonylureas (ie, glipizide) and biguanides (ie, metformin), have also been used in the treatment of diabetes in people and cats, but are only effective in patients that have NIDDM [45]. Glipizide, the most commonly used oral hypoglycemic in cats, directly stimulates beta cells to secrete insulin. This medication requires that the pancreatic beta cells have some remaining secretory capacity to be effective. Metformin has no direct effect on beta cells, but rather exerts its effects by enhancing insulin sensitivity in hepatic and peripheral tissues, which, in turn, increases the insulin's ability to transport glucose across cell membranes, inhibits hepatic gluconeogenesis and glycogenolysis, and decreases glucose absorption in the gastrointestinal tract [48]. Because this medication does not stimulate insulin production or release, it is unlikely to cause hypoglycemia [34,48]. Because the type of diabetes ferrets are likely to be afflicted with is undetermined at this time, it is questionable whether these medications would be of any benefit to diabetic ferrets.

Recently, the role of carbohydrates in the carnivore diet and the management of diabetes has come under investigation. It is believed that felines, as pure carnivores, are not adapted to metabolize carbohydrates effectively and are naturally more resistant to the effects of insulin [49]. Ferrets are also pure carnivores and may have a similar ineffective mechanism for metabolizing carbohydrates. Studies in diabetic cats have demonstrated that cats fed low carbohydrate-high protein diets have better glycemic control, require less insulin, and have increased rates of diabetic remission [47].

Serial blood glucose curves can be used to monitor response to therapy. Insulin efficacy and duration, time of peak effect, and glucose nadirs can be assessed. However, the multiple venipunctures required to obtain a glucose curve are often not practical in ferrets because they have small veins and have a smaller volume of blood, compared with cats. As with cats, the stress or refusal of food during hospitalization may also artificially alter the blood glucose concentration. To circumvent this problem, home monitoring has become more popular in the management of diabetic cats. At the authors' practice, one owner was able to use a lancet normally used for people on her ferret's foot pads to check the ferret's blood glucose daily. However, according to the owner's observation, over time the foot pads became calloused and it became increasingly difficult to obtain an adequate blood sample. Portable glucometers can differ greatly in performance and validation for use in ferrets is recommended.

Because the pathophysiology of diabetes is not fully understood in ferrets, treatment recommendations should be made cautiously. Owners with diabetic ferrets should be advised that these ferrets can be very difficult to regulate tightly because of the variable response to exogenous insulin. In the authors' practice, one ferret would fluctuate between episodes of hyperglycemia and hypoglycemia, regardless of administration of insulin. One possible explanation for this finding was the possible development of a coexisting insulinoma with erratic insulin release. Because of these circumstances, spontaneous diabetes usually has a guarded-to-poor prognosis.

Summary

Pancreatic endocrinopathies, especially insulinomas, are a common finding in ferrets. Surgical resection remains the treatment of choice for insulinomas because it can provide longer disease-free intervals and survival times. Because of the high rate of metastasis, owners should be advised that treatment is rarely curative and is aimed at controlling the clinical signs of hypoglycemia by stopping or slowing the progression of the insulinoma. Although less common, diabetes mellitus can occur is ferrets, but it is often a postsurgical sequela to insulinoma resection. Current advancements in diabetes management can be applied to ferrets with diabetes mellitus.

References

[1] Willams BH, Weiss CA. Ferret neoplasia. In: Quesenberry KE, Carpenter JW, editors. Ferrets, rabbits, and rodents: clinical medicine. 2nd edition. St. Louis (MO): Saunders; 2003. p. 91–106.

[2] Lewington JH. Endocrine diseases. In: Lewington JH, editor. Ferret husbandry, medicine & surgery. Edinburgh (IN): Elsevier Science Limited; 2002. p. 211–22.

[3] Eatwell K. Two unusual tumours in a ferret (Mustela putorius furo). J Small Anim Pract 2004;45(9):454–9.

[4] Lloyd CG, Lewis WG. Two cases of pancreatic neoplasia in British ferrets (Mustela putorius furo). J Small Anim Pract 2004;45(11):558–62.

[5] Lair S, Barker IK, Mehren KG, et al. Epidemiology of neoplasia in captive black-footed ferrets (Mustela nigripes), 1986–1996. J Zoo Wildl Med 2002;33(3):204–13.

[6] Lewington JH. Nutrition. In: Lewington JH, editor. Ferret husbandry, medicine & surgery. Edinburgh (IN): Elsevier Science Limited; 2002. p. 54–74.

[7] Evans HE, An NQ. Anatomy of the ferret. In: Fox JD, editor. Biology and diseases of the ferret. 2nd edition. Baltimore (MD): Williams &Wilkins; 1998. p. 19–70.

[8] Jenkins JR. Ferret metabolic testing. In: Fudge AM, editor. Laboratory medicine: avian and exotic pets. Philadelphia: WB Saunders; 2000. p. 305–9.

[9] Lurye JC, Behrend EN. Endocrine tumors. Vet Clin North Am Small Anim Pract 2001; 33(5):1083–110.

[10] Guyton AC, Hall JE. Insulin, glucagon, and diabetes mellitus. In: Textbook of medical physiology. 10th edition. Philadelphia: WB Saunders; 2000. p. 884–97.

[11] Fox JG, Marini RP. Diseases of the endocrine system. In: Fox JD, editor. Biology and diseases of the ferret. 2nd edition. Baltimore (MD): Williams &Wilkins; 1998. p. 291–306.

[12] Whary MK, Andrew PLR. Physiology of the ferret. In: Fox JD, editor. Biology and diseases of the ferret. 2nd edition. Baltimore (MD): Williams &Wilkins; 1998. p. 103–48.

[13] Hoefer HL, Patnaik AK, Lewis AD. Pancreatic adenocarcinoma with metastasis in two ferrets. J Am Vet Med Assoc 1992;201(3):466–7.

[14] Li X, Fox JG, Padrid PA. Neoplastic diseases in ferrets: 574 cases (1968–1997). J Am Vet Med Assoc 1998;212(9):1402–6.

[15] Jergens AE, Shaw DP. Hyperinsulinism and hypoglycemia associated with pancreatic islet cell tumor in a ferret. J Am Vet Med Assoc 1989;94(2):269–71.

[16] Luttgen PJ, Storts RW, Rogers KS, et al. Insulinoma in a ferret. J Am Vet Med Assoc 1986; 189(8):920–1.

[17] Caplan ER, Peterson ME, Mullen HS, et al. Diagnosis and treatment of insulin-secreting pancreatic islet cell tumors in ferrets: 57 cases (1986–1994). J Am Vet Med Assoc 1996; 209(10):1741–5.

[18] Quesenberry KE, Rosenthal KL. Endocrine diseases. In: Quesenberry KE, Carpenter JW, editors. Ferrets, rabbits, and rodents: clinical medicine and surgery. 2nd edition. St. Louis (MO): Saunders; 2003. p. 79–90.

[19] Fix AS, Harms CA. Immunocytochemistry of pancreatic endocrine tumors in three domestic ferrets (Mustela putorius furo). Vet Pathol 1990;27:199–201.

[20] Antinoff N, Hahn K. Ferret oncology: diseases, diagnostics, and therapeutics. Vet Clin North Am Exot Anim Pract 2004;7(3):579–625.

[21] Elie MS, Zerbe CA. Insulinoma in dogs, cats, and ferrets. Compendium on Continuing Education for the Practicing Veterinarian 1995;17(1):51–9.

[22] Marini RP, Ryden EB, Rosenblad BS, et al. Functional islet cell tumor in six ferrets. J Am Vet Med Assoc 1993;202(3):430–4.

[23] Lumeij JT, van der Hage MH, Dorrestein GM, et al. Hypoglycaemia due to a functional pancreatic islet cell tumour (insulinoma) in a ferret (Mustela putorius furo). Vet Rec 1987;120: 129–30.

[24] Meleo KA, Caplan ER. Treatment of insulinoma in the dog, cat, and ferret. In: Bonagura JD, editor. Current veterinary therapy XIII. Philadelphia: WB Saunders; 1999. p. 357–61.

[25] Ehrhart N, Withrow SJ, Ehrhart EJ, et al. Pancreatic beta cell tumor in ferrets: 20 cases (1986–1994). J Am Vet Med Assoc 1996;209(10):1737–40.

[26] Rosenthal KL. Ferret and rabbit endocrine disease diagnosis. In: Fudge AM, editor. Laboratory medicine: avian and exotic pets. Philadelphia: WB Saunders; 2000. p. 319–24.

[27] Mann FA, Stockham SL, Freeman MB, et al. Reference intervals for insulin concentrations and insulin: glucose ratios in the serum of ferrets. Journal of Small Exotic Animal Medicine 1993;2(2):79–83.

[28] Antinoff N. Neoplasia in ferrets. In: Bonagura JD, editor. Current veterinary therapy XIII. Philadelphia: WB Saunders; 1999. p. 1149–52.

[29] Elliott DA, Nelson RW, Feldman EC, et al. Glycosylated hemoglobin concentrations in the blood of healthy dogs and dogs with naturally developing diabetes mellitus, pancreatic beta-cell neoplasia, hyperadrenocorticism, and anemia. J Am Vet Med Assoc 1997;211(6):723–7.

[30] Polton GA, White RN, Brearley MJ, et al. Improved survival in a retrospective cohort of 28 dogs with insulinoma. J Small Anim Pract 2007;48:151–6.

[31] Andrews GA, Myers NC. Immunohistochemistry of pancreatic islet cell tumors in the ferret (Mustela putorius furo). Vet Pathol 1997;34(5):387–93.

[32] Weiss CA, Willams BH, Scott MV. Insulinoma in the ferret: clinical findings and treatment comparison of 66 cases. J Am Anim Hosp Assoc 1998;34(6):471–5.

[33] Fingeroth JM, Smeak DD. Intravenous methylene blue infusion for intraoperative identification of pancreatic islet-cell tumors in dogs. Part II: clinical trials and results in four dogs. J Am Anim Hosp Assoc 1988;24(2):175–82.

[34] Plumb DC. Plumb's veterinary drug handbook. 5th edition. Stockholm (WI): Blackwell; 2005.

[35] Exotic animal formulary. In: Carpenter JW, editor. 3rd edition. Philadelphia: WB Saunders; 2004.

[36] Usukura M, Yoneda T, Oda N, et al. Medical treatment of benign insulinoma using octreotide LAR: a case report. Endocr J 2007;54(1):95–101.

[37] Rosenthal KL. Feeding the hypoglycemic ferret. In: Proceedings for North American Veterinary Conference. Orlando (FL): 2006. p. 1766.

[38] Blackwood L. Multiple endocrine neoplasia syndromes (MEN) in humans and animals. In: Proceedings for the 15th ECVIM-CA Congress. Glasgow (UK): 2005. Available at: http://www.vin.com/Members/Proceedings/Proceedings.plx?CID=ECVIM2005%. Accessed February 15, 2007.

[39] Carpenter JW, Novilla MN. Diabetes mellitus in a black-footed ferret. J Am Vet Med Assoc 1977;171(9):890–3.

[40] Hillyer E. Ferret endocrinology. In: Kirk RW, Bonagura JD, editors. Current veterinary therapy XI: small animal practice. Philadelphia: WB Saunders; 1992. p. 1185–8.

[41] Benoit-Biancamano MO, Morin M, Langlois I. Histopathologic lesions of diabetes mellitus in a domestic ferret. Can Vet J 2005;46:895–7.

[42] Hackendahl N, Schaer M. Insulin resistance in diabetic patients: mechanisms and classifications. Compendium on Continuing Education for the Practicing Veterinarian 2006;28(4): 262–70.

[43] Stephen D. White. Cutaneous paraneoplastic syndromes. In: Proceedings from the American College of Veterinary Internal Medicine Forum. Baltimore (MD): 2005. Available at: http://www.vin.com/Members/Proceedings/Proceedings.plx?CID=ACVIM2005&; PID=pr09509&Print=1&O=VIN. Accessed February 15, 2007.

[44] Johnson-Delaney CA. Ferret endocrinopathies. In: Proceedings from the Atlantic Coast Veterinary Conference. Atlantic City (NJ): 2005. Available at: http://www.vin.com/Members/

Proceedings/Proceedings.plx?CID=acvc2005&;PID=pr10684&O=VIN. Accessed February 15, 2007.

[45] Nelson RW. Endocrine disorders. In: Nelson RW, Couto CG, editors. Small animal internal medicine. 3rd edition. St. Louis (MO): Mosby; 2003. p. 729–77.

[46] Weaver KE, Rozanski EA, Mahony OM, et al. Use of glargine and lente insulins in cats with diabetes mellitus. J Vet Intern Med 2006;20:234–8.

[47] Rand JS, Marshall RD. Diabetes mellitus in cats. Vet Clin North Am Small Anim Pract 2005;35:211–24.

[48] Nelson R, Spann D, Elliott D, et al. Evaluation of the oral antihyperglycemic drug metformin in normal and diabetic cats. J Vet Intern Med 2004;18:18–24.

[49] Slingerland LI, Robben JH, van Haeften TW, et al. Insulin sensitivity and beta-cell function in healthy cats: assessment with the use of the hyperglycemic glucose clamp. Horm Metab Res 2007;39(5):341–6.

VETERINARY
CLINICS
Exotic Animal Practice

ELSEVIER
SAUNDERS

Vet Clin Exot Anim 11 (2008) 125–137

Adrenal Gland Disease in Ferrets

Elisabeth Simone-Freilicher, DVM, DABVP–Avian

Avian and Exotic Medicine Department, Veterinary Medical Center of Long Island,
75 Sunrise Highway, West Islip, NY 11795, USA

Adrenal gland disease has been recognized in ferrets for nearly 20 years in the United States [1,2]. The prevalence of the disease appears to be increasing; 70% of pet ferrets in the United States were estimated to be affected in 2003, compared with 30% in 1993 [3]. It is important for the practitioner to understand the anatomy and physiology of the adrenal gland, to assess current and emerging treatment options, and to make appropriate recommendations tailored to the individual patient.

Anatomy and physiology

The adrenal glands are located adjacent to the cranial borders of the right and left kidneys, often entirely embedded in fat, and covered by a thin peritoneum [3–5]. The adrenal cortex is made up of a zona glomerulosa, fasciculata, and reticularis, as in domestic mammals, and a zona intermedia and juxtamedullaris [6]. The right adrenal gland is larger and more elongated than the left, and both glands may increase in mass during late proestrus or full estrus in the female ferret [3,6]. The left adrenal gland is usually 2 to 3 mm wide, up to 6 to 8 mm long, and is situated left of the abdominal aorta, and caudal to the cranial mesenteric artery [3,4]. The right adrenal gland is usually 8 to 11 mm long, and located more cranially than the left adrenal gland [3]. The elongated right adrenal gland lies ventral to the vena cava under the caudate lobe of the liver, may curve to the right around the vena cava, and may even encompass the dorsal side of the vessel [1,3,4]. Fascia may also adhere the right adrenal gland to the vena cava [7]. Because of its more cranial location, the right adrenal gland may be more difficult to palpate than the left [1]. Individual variations of the blood supply exist, but, in general, a branch of the aorta supplies the cranial pole, branches from the renal artery supply the caudal pole, and an additional

E-mail address: freilicherdvm@aol.com

branch from the aorta supplies the left adrenal gland [5]. The phrenicoabdo-
minal vein is found on the ventral surface of the gland, coursing from lateral
to medial [4]. In ferrets with adrenal gland disease, the adrenal glands may
be grossly enlarged and cystic, or they may extend into adjacent tissue, including the caudal vena cava [8]. Adjacent histologically normal accessory
adrenal tissue may also be found [5,9].

As in other mammals, the adrenal gland secretes cortisol, and plasma cortisol concentrations are affected by corticotropin stimulation and dexamethasone suppression testing. Corticotropin increases cortisol for 30 to 60
minutes; dexamethasone decreases cortisol for 1 to 5 hours [6]. Plasma cortisol is not increased in ferrets with adrenal gland disease, although urinary
cortisol levels may rise relative to urinary creatinine [2,6]. The adrenocortical zona reticularis secretes sex hormones, including estradiol, 17-hydroxy-
progesterone, dehydroepiandrosterone, and androstenedione, and it is this
layer that is affected by adrenal gland disease [10].

Proposed etiology

The exact cause of the adrenal gland changes that lead to adrenal gland disease in ferrets is unknown [1]. The disease is more prevalent in ferrets in the
United States than in Europe or Australia, possibly because of the small
founder population and closed colonies of large breeders [11]. Ferrets outside
the United States are typically less inbred, and experience husbandry conditions (including diet and photoperiod) similar to the environmental pressures
under which they evolved. A study of European ferrets demonstrated a correlation between age at sterilization and age at onset of adrenal gland disease
[10]. It is believed that the early oophorohysterectomies and neutering of ferrets in the United States (typically between 4 and 6 weeks of age) may be a contributing factor in the development of adrenal gland disease [2–4,10]. This
theory is supported by studies in mice, which show that early sterilization
can result in adrenal neoplasia or adrenocortical nodular hyperplasia arising
from undifferentiated gonadal cells incorporated into the adrenal capsule during embryologic development [1,2]. The hypothalamus of the sterilized ferret
continues to secrete gonadotropin-releasing hormone (GnRH), stimulating
the pituitary gland, which in turn secretes luteinizing hormone (LH) and follicle-stimulating hormone [3]. If ferrets similarly incorporate gonadal cells into
the adrenal gland, LH and follicle-stimulating hormone will stimulate these
and the zona reticularis, resulting in increased secretion of sex hormones
[2,3,12]. The absence of the normal gonadal secretion of estrogens and androgens results in a lack of negative feedback on the hypothalamus, causing continuous release of GnRH and continuous stimulation of the hormonal cascade
[3,4]. In mice, the elevated levels of circulating LH are considered a prerequisite
for adrenal neoplastic changes [13].

The effects of early sterilization combined with the artificially prolonged
photoperiod experienced by indoor pet ferrets are believed to predispose

ferrets in the United States to adrenal gland disease [3,14,15]. Ferrets are considered highly sensitive to photoperiod, as is demonstrated by the hormonal cycling of unspayed female ferrets in response to a prolonged photoperiod [3]. Ferrets kept at light cycles longer than 8 hours have been reported to have increased GnRH and LH production [16]. It is thought that ferrets experiencing artificially prolonged photoperiods may become deficient in melatonin, a hormone produced by the pineal gland during dark hours [3].

It has also been proposed that the progression of adrenal gland tumors is not under pituitary control, but rather under the control of an abnormal tumor suppressor gene, because the pituitary of affected ferrets has a low density of gonadotropin-positive cells [17]. Adrenal gland neoplasia may have a genetic component, because it has been shown that the protein marker GATA-4 is expressed in cases of ferret adrenocortical adenomas and carcinomas, but is not present in cases of adrenal hyperplasia [12,17,18]. In humans, multiple endocrine neoplasias (as are common in ferrets) nearly always have a genetic cause; research is currently ongoing to determine whether mutations in similar genes in ferrets can be identified in neoplastic tissue. Early sterilization may play an initiating role by causing an LH surge, which causes the initial hyperactivity of the adrenal cortex, resulting in early-sterilized ferrets with the same seasonal hormonal levels as intact ferrets [17]. Preliminary research into inducing a hormonal state similar to breeding for these ferrets by administering Lupron at the time of the ferrets' first breeding season is promising [17].

Pathophysiology

Adrenal gland disease in ferrets is caused by adrenocortical adenoma (16%), hyperplasia (56%), or adenocarcinoma (26%), causing a release of excess sex hormones, particularly estradiol [1–3,16]. Of these, epithelial adenomas are the most common, and the left adrenal seems to be affected more commonly [1,9,19]. A mixed adenocarcinoma consisting of epithelial cells and spindles cells has also been reported, and is associated with decreased survival time and decreased disease-free interval [19]. A particularly malignant adrenal cortical carcinoma with myxoid differentiation has also been described [12]. Grossly affected glands may be cystic, discolored, enlarged, or irregular [20]. Additionally, atrophy, hyperplasia, or neoplasia of the contralateral gland may occur [2].

Plasma cortisol concentrations are usually not increased in ferrets with adrenal gland disease; however, estradiol, 17-hydroxyprogesterone, or androstenedione are most commonly elevated [2,6,14,21]. Dehydroepiandrosterone sulfate may also be elevated [2,16]. High levels of estrogen are thought to contribute to vulvar enlargement in female ferrets, and squamous metaplasia of the prostatic ducts and cystic prostatic disease in male ferrets [2,12]. Mild to pyogranulomatous inflammation of the prostate may also occur in these ferrets [22]. Increased androgen levels may slow the hair follicle growth phase, resulting in hair loss [2].

Infrequently, other organ changes may occur, including lymphocyte depletion of lymph nodes, and irregularly arranged dermal collagen [2]. Adrenal tumors rarely metastasize; however, carcinoma metastasis to the lungs or liver does occur infrequently [1,12]. Local invasion of the liver or adjacent viscera can occur, particularly by a right adrenal carcinoma [2,9]. Tumor necrosis, rupture, and loss of quality of life can all occur [11].

Signalment

Ferrets of either sex can be affected by adrenal gland disease. Some investigators suspect a bias in reporting of female ferrets, because many ferret owners recognize an enlarged vulva as requiring medical attention [1,2]. Other studies show no difference in prevalence between the sexes [9,10]. Reported ages range from 8 months to 9 years, although the average age is 3.5 to 4.5 years [3].

Signs

Progressive alopecia with ease of epilation is the primary clinical sign of ferret adrenal gland disease, occurring in more than 90% of cases [1–3,9]. Often, the hair loss progresses from the tail, rump, or flanks to the dorsum, lateral flanks, and ventrum (Fig. 1) [1,2]. Initially, hair loss may occur during the spring and may continue to progress, or seem to resolve with hair regrowth in the fall [1,2]. In one report, pruritis occurred in approximately 40% of ferrets, with or without hair loss, and it can be intense and unresponsive to antihistamines or steroids [9,23]. Lethargy, muscle atrophy, and strong odor can also occur [3,9]. More than 70% of female ferrets with adrenal gland disease display vulvar swelling (Fig. 2), with occasional mucoid discharge consistent with vaginitis and stump pyometra [1,3]. Male ferrets can show prostatic enlargement with associated periurethral cysts, which may cause narrowing of the urethra, resulting in dysuria, strangury, or complete blockage [1–3]. Tenesmus is also reported by owners [12], either as a result of prostatic enlargement or because of involuntary defecation during strangury. Mammary gland enlargement may occur in female ferrets, and is infrequently reported in male ferrets, and sexual aggression is occasionally reported in either sex [2,12]. Sexual aggression in male ferrets has been associated with adrenocortical carcinoma [2]. Complete urinary blockage in male ferrets is an emergency, as in other species, because it may result in metabolic derangements that are life-threatening [1].

Enlarged adrenal glands may be detectable on palpation [4]. The left adrenal gland is more often affected, and is more readily palpable than the right [2].

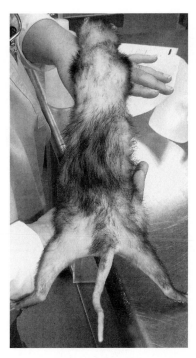

Fig. 1. Alopecia in a ferret with adrenal gland disease. Note the hair loss on the tail, legs, rump, and shoulders, and thinning hair coat over the dorsum. This ferret also had a characteristically strong scent.

Diagnostic testing

History, clinical signs, and response to hormone therapy may form the basis of a presumptive diagnosis in many cases. Testing for elevations of all three sex hormones (estradiol, androstenedione, and 17-hydroxyproges-terone) may provide better sensitivity for identifying adrenal gland disease then testing of a single hormone [21].

Ultrasound may be of equal, or better, diagnostic value than hormonal panels, according to some investigators [6]. If surgery is desired, ultrasonog-raphy can also provide identification of the affected gland, as well as size, architecture, neovascularization, and concurrent disease [1,14]. A prominent uterus, a uterine stump, or an enlarged prostate may also be detected [24]. An absence of periglandular fat between the adrenal gland and the large vessels, or deviation or compression of the large vessels, may indicate nonre-sectability or malignancy [24]. Abnormal adrenal glands have a rounded appearance, increased size of either pole (>3.9 mm), increased echogenicity or heterogeneity, or mineralization [25]. Hyperplasia or adrenal adenomas may appear ultrasonographically normal [24]. Accessory adrenal tissue can-not always be identified on ultrasound [26]. Definitive diagnosis can be

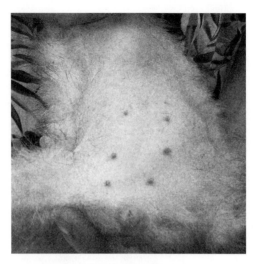

Fig. 2. Enlarged vulva and mammaries in a female ferret with adrenal gland disease. Alopecia over the abdomen is also present.

achieved most accurately by histopathology of samples obtained by adrenalectomy or surgical biopsy [1].

Other clinical pathology

Complete blood count and biochemical profiles are usually unremarkable in ferrets with adrenal gland disease [1]. A nonregenerative anemia, thrombocytopenia, and hypoglycemia have also been reported occasionally in ferrets with adrenal gland disease [2,23]. Pancytopenia may be seen, similar to that of ferrets with estrogen-induced bone marrow suppression [1]. Profound anemia from estrogen suppression of bone marrow may occur in ferrets with adrenal gland disease, but is reportedly rare [7]. Plasma concentrations of cortisol, corticotropin, and α-melanocyte–stimulating hormone are not elevated in ferrets with adrenal gland disease; however, urine cortisol/creatinine ratio may be elevated, and is resistant to dexamethasone suppression [1,2,27,28].

Radiography generally is not useful for detecting adrenal mineralization or adrenal masses, because the masses rarely create a detectable mass effect [1,2].

Differential diagnosis

Differential diagnoses include ovarian remnant in spayed female ferrets and estrus in intact female ferrets, both of which are much less common than adrenal gland disease [2,9]. Estradiol may be elevated in each condition; however, in female ferrets, androgens will only be elevated with adrenal gland disease [1]. In intact female ferrets, or those with ovarian remnants, treatment with 1000 U of human chorionic gonadotropin+ repeated 2 weeks apart will reduce vulva size [7]. Ultrasonography may help differentiate between these conditions, or exploratory surgery may be required [1].

Treatment

Male ferrets presenting as an emergency for urinary blockage require immediate attention and treatment. A full bladder or enlarged or cystic prostate can be palpated (Fig. 3), and fluid-filled cysts can be identified ultrasonographically and differentiated from calculi [7]. The cysts can be aspirated percutaneously to help relieve the blockage. Fluid should be submitted for culture and sensitivity when possible, because the prostatic tissue may be sterile, or may be infected and require aggressive antibiotic therapy [1,8]. A 3.5F or urinary catheter or a 3.0 ferret catheter (ProVet, Kansas City, Missouri) should be placed to relieve the blockage (Fig. 4), and may be kept in place for 1 to 2 days, which is usually sufficient to relieve the obstruction [1,7,20]. Most ferrets require isoflurane anesthesia, and magnifying loops may facilitate visualization of the urethral opening [7,20]. Cystocentesis should be avoided if possible because of the risk of bladder rupture [7]. Hormonal or surgical treatment of the adrenal gland should be initiated, and in-house chemistry should be performed to assess for the presence of electrolyte imbalance, which may require treatment [7]. A testosterone blocker may be added to the treatment to decrease prostatic size more quickly [14]. Large infected cysts may require surgical management, including drainage, debulking, marsupialization, or omentalization [20].

Surgical excision or debulking of the affected gland is the preferred treatment for ferrets that are suitable surgical candidates [1,4,9]. Surgical management also allows direct visualization of other potentially diseased

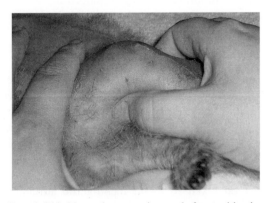

Fig. 3. Severely distended bladder and prostate in a male ferret with adrenal gland disease.

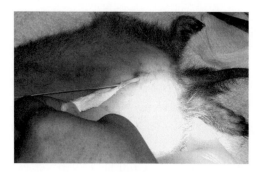

Fig. 4. Catheter placement in a male ferret with urethral obstructive impingement from prostatomegaly. Gauze is hooked over the curved tip of the penis to maintain the penis outside of the prepuce, and the urethra is visible at the ventral tip.

organs, particularly the pancreas and abdominal lymph nodes, which are commonly affected by insulinoma and lymphosarcoma, respectively [1].

Before surgery, the ferret should be fasted for approximately 4 hours [7]. Blood glucose should be monitored during this time, and ferrets with insulinoma should receive intravenous dextrose administration in fluids [7].

A ventral midline incision should be made beginning 1 to 2 cm caudal to the xiphoid toward the midabdomen, extended sufficiently to permit examination of the abdominal organs [4]. In addition to the pancreas and intestinal lymph nodes, other organs such as the liver, kidneys, and spleen should be examined and biopsied as appropriate [7]. Incidental gastrointestinal foreign bodies may also be identified and addressed [4]. In male ferrets, the prostate should be palpated for the presence of enlargement and cysts, whereas in female ferrets, the ovarian and uterine stumps should be inspected [4]. Following abdominal exploratory, both adrenal glands should be examined and compared, because bilateral adrenal gland disease can be present [1]. Visibility may be improved by exteriorizing the spleen and small intestine, which should then be protected with a laparotomy sponge soaked with warmed saline solution [20]. Left adrenalectomy is simple to perform; however, removal of the right adrenal gland can be more challenging [7]. Ultrasonography before surgery to identify the affected gland or glands can help prepare owners for the relative risk of the surgery and the prognosis for complete removal of the lesion.

The left adrenal gland is located cranial to the left kidney, and may be dissected free from adipose tissue while ligating the small vessels attached to it [7]. A combination of sharp and blunt dissection and instruments, including microsurgical forceps, mosquito hemostats, and moistened cotton-tipped applicators, can all be helpful for this delicate procedure [4]. Generally, three to four vessels will be located, including both sides of the phrenicolumbar vein and feeder branches from the aorta and renal artery [5,20]. Care must be taken to avoid nicking the adrenal gland, because when the gland is diseased, it may be vascular and bleeding can be difficult to control [20]. Once all adrenal vessels are exposed, hemostasis may be provided, using cautery or hemostatic clips [4,20].

Right adrenalectomy is considered more challenging because of its frequently found fascial attachment to the vena cava, and occasional vascular invasion [4,7]. Damage to the vena cava can cause severe hemorrhage; debulking the right adrenal gland is often a preferred option [7]. However, this approach leaves hormone-secreting tissue still present in the ferret, and the tumor may continue to grow and produce clinical signs [7]. Fortunately, the right adrenal is reported to require removal in only 15% to 20% of cases [4]. The hepatorenal ligament may be resected and used to retract the caudate lobe of the liver, permitting better visualization of the gland and its relationship to the vena cava [4]. Magnifying loops may also facilitate visualization. If invasion has not occurred, small tumors can be partially freed from the vena cava with gentle dissection, and a hemostatic clip placed between the vessel and the gland, permitting resection [4]. In cases of caval invasion, a small, double-angled vascular clamp, such as a neonatal Satinsky clamp or DeBakey cardiovascular clamp, may be used to occlude the vessel during removal [4,20]. If a nick occurs in the vena cava, hemostatic gel and 5 minutes of pressure may be used to control hemorrhage [20]. A larger defect in the vessel may be repaired using 8-0, 9-0, or 10-0 nylon on a small atraumatic needle in a simple continuous pattern [4,20]. A gelatin sponge, such as Surgicel (Johnson and Johnson, Somerville, New Jersey) or Gelfoam (Pharmacia and Upjohn, Kalamazoo, Michigan) may be placed over the suture line to help restrict mild oozing [4,20]. If a vena cava laceration cannot be repaired, it may require ligation. Ligation should be avoided if possible, because up to 30% of ferrets can undergo acute renal failure following vena cava ligation [20]. Alternately, the gland can be partially debulked, or the capsule incised and the gland shelled out from the capsule. However, if right glandular tissue is left behind, the adrenal gland disease can recur, including the more aggressive adenocarcinoma, which may invade the vena cava or caudate liver lobe [20]. Laser surgery, cryosurgery, and radiosurgical ablation of the gland have all been reported; however, thermal damage to the vena cava is a concern, and histologic examination of the affected gland is not possible [4].

Postsurgically, the ferret should receive supportive care and analgesia for 2 to 3 days [20]. Postoperative glucocorticoid replacement is usually not necessary, because excess cortisol secretion is not part of this disease syndrome [7]. However, if the ferret seems particularly lethargic after surgery, with no other clinical signs or apparent reason, dexamethasone sodium phosphate (2–4 mg/kg IV) can be administered [7]. Packed cell volume, blood glucose, and blood pressure should also be monitored and addressed as needed [4]. Because of the risk of recurrent malignancy, total adrenalectomy is preferred by some practitioners; these ferrets should receive a tapering prednisone dose postsurgically (0.1–0.5 mg/kg every 12–24 hours) [20].

Partial or subtotal adrenalectomy yields a good prognosis where there is no encroachment into the caudal vena cava [2]. Subtotal bilateral adrenalectomy has been reported to yield a mortality rate of 2% to 13% [4,9]. Recurrence after unilateral adrenalectomy has been reported at 17% [15]. When debulking is used, survival may be improved by concurrent use of hormone suppression therapy [17]. Clinical signs usually resolve within 2 to 4 weeks of surgery, and may recur in some ferrets within 11 to 24 months [4,9].

Medical management is palliative only, and relieves clinical signs without inhibiting the growth of the tumor [1]. Medical treatment may be of benefit to older or medically compromised ferrets, or those for which surgery is not an option [11]. Few controlled clinical trials or toxicity studies exist, and none of these medications are labeled for use in ferrets [14].

GnRH agonists act by down-regulating gonadotropin receptors in the pituitary [1,14]. The GnRH agonist most commonly used in ferrets is leuprolide acetate, 100 to 150 mcg/kg per month [16]. (Lupron Depot, TAP Pharmaceuticals, Lake Forest, Illinois). Initially, the agonist hyperstimulates GnRH receptors, resulting in a negative feedback that down-regulates GnRH receptors, and the production of gonadotropin, which stimulates adrenal production of steroids [14,29]. In most ferrets, most clinical signs resolve within 6 to 8 weeks, although some ferrets retain a thin pelage or poor regrowth of tail hair [16]. Lupron 30-day formulation has been shown to result in sex steroid suppression in intact ferrets for 30 days, and the 3-month formulation has been shown to cause suppression in most ferrets for 60 to 90 days [14,17]. Studies in ferrets with adrenal gland disease show suppression of estradiol, androstenedione, dihydroepiandrosterone, and 17-hydroxyprogesterone for 1 to 3 months, without adverse affects [16]. Anecdotal evidence suggests the 4-month Lupron depot does not relieve clinical signs for 4 months [14]. Individual variations in duration of effectiveness are thought to be related to variations in dose and individual sensitivity, or variations in response by adrenal hyperplasia, adenoma, or adenocarcinoma [16].

Deslorelin acetate (Suprelorin, Peptech Animal Health, North Ryde, Australia) is another synthetic GnRH analog that is placed as a slow-release implant, and may decrease clinical signs and suppress sex hormone concentrations [15]. One study of a 3-mg slow-release deslorelin implant showed a decrease in clinical signs and plasma hormone concentrations for 8 to 20 months [11]. No adverse effects were noted in this study, and tumor growth was not inhibited [11].

Aromatase inhibitors inhibit the final catalyzing enzyme in estrogen production [1]. Of these, Anastrozole at 0.1 mg/kg by mouth every 24 hours (Arimidex, AstraZeneca Pharmaceuticals, Wilmington, Delaware) may be of use in ferrets with prostatic disease associated with high estradiol levels [14].

Androgen blockers have also been used in ferrets, and may be particularly effective in male ferrets with prostatic disease secondary to adrenal gland disease [14]. Bicalutamide (Casodex, AstraZeneca Pharmaceuticals, Wilmington, Delaware) is dosed at 5 mg/kg by mouth every 24 hours, and must be given with an antigonadotropin medication (such as Lupron), because it can increase levels of testosterone and estradiol when used alone [14]. Flutamide (Eulexin, Schering Corporation, Kenilworth, New Jersey) has also been suggested for use in ferrets; however, it has been associated with increases in mammary tumors in rats, and further investigation of the use of this drug in ferrets is recommended [14].

Melatonin has been reported to cause short-term suppression of sex hormones and clinical signs, including fur loss, pruritis, and decrease in vulva and prostate size [15,17]. One small study has shown significant decrease in serum estradiol and prolactin following the use of oral melatonin for 4 to 8 months [15]. Androsterone and 17-hydroxyprogesterone also decreased, but not significantly [15]. However, after 12 months of oral treatment, estradiol, androsterone, and 17-hydroxyprogesterone levels increased, and clinical signs recurred [15]. Endogenous melatonin is synthesized in the pineal gland from serotonin [15]. Exogenous melatonin has been used in mink to promote thick fur growth; studies suggest that melatonin regulates prolactin, which has receptors in the skin and adrenal gland [15]. In humans, it is contraindicated in patients with hepatic insufficiency, and should be used with caution in cases of renal impairment [30]. No adverse affects were reported in the oral melatonin study, and tumor growth was not affected [14,15]. Oral melatonin may be compounded and given at 0.5 to 1.0 mg/day, preferably 8 hours after sunrise; melatonin implants have also been used [14,17] (Ferretonin, Melatek, Fort Collins, Colorado).

Mitotane (Lysodren, Anabolic, Irvine, California) has been used as a form of cytotoxic debulking of the adrenal glands, with fair to poor results described in ferrets [7,9]. In dogs, it is known to cause severe progressive necrosis of the zona reticularis and fasciculate [31]. Mitotane can be compounded to 50 mg capsules, and given 50 mg per ferret by mouth every 24 hours for 1 week, followed by 50 mg by mouth two to three times per week [31]. However, because it is not specific to the sex hormone–producing cells of the zona reticularis, it may decrease cortisol production and trigger hypoglycemia when concurrent insulinoma is present [9,14]. Pulsing the therapy one to two times per week may be better tolerated; however, bioavailability and pharmacologic studies are needed [14]. Mitotane can exacerbate pre-existing liver disease, and may also increase the hepatic metabolism of some medications; therefore, monitoring of liver enzymes is recommended [31]. When mitotane does achieve resolution of clinical signs, signs may recur and are rarely suppressed by a second course of this treatment [7]. Other adverse effects may include anorexia, vomiting, diarrhea, and poorly responsive hypoglycemia when concurrent insulinoma is present [9].

Summary

Adrenal gland disease affects approximately 70% of pet ferrets in the United States. It is important for the ferret practitioner to be familiar with the pathophysiology and proposed causes of the disease to make informed recommendations to clients owning unaffected animals. An understanding of the medical and surgical options for treating adrenal gland disease, along with their advantages and disadvantages, is necessary to make appropriate recommendations to clients while additional treatment modalities are being developed, and to evaluate currently available and future treatment options.

References

[1] Quesenberry KE, Rosenthal KL. Endocrine diseases. In: Quesenberry KE, Carpenter JW, editors. Ferrets, rabbits, and rodents: clinical medicine and surgery. Philadelphia: Saunders; 2004. p. 121–34.

[2] Fox JG, Marini RP. Diseases of the endocrine system. In: Fox JG, editor. Biology and diseases of the ferret. 2nd edition. New York: Lippincott Williams and Wilkins; 1998. p. 291–305.

[3] Lewington J. Ferrets. In: O'Malley B, editor. Clinical anatomy and physiology of exotic species. New York: Elsevier Limited; 2005. p. 236–61.

[4] Ludwig L, Aiken S. Soft tissue surgery. In: Quesenberry KE, Carpenter JW, editors. Ferrets, rabbits, and rodents: clinical medicine and surgery. Philadelphia: Saunders; 2004. p. 121–34.

[5] Evans HE, An NQ. Anatomy of the ferret. In: Fox JG, editor. Biology and diseases of the ferret. 2nd edition. New York: Lippincott Williams and Wilkins; 1998. p. 19–69.

[6] Whary MT, Andrews PLR. Physiology of the ferret. In: Fox JG, editor. Biology and diseases of the ferret. 2nd edition. New York: Lippincott Williams and Wilkins; 1998. p. 103–48.

[7] Rosenthal KL, Peterson ME. Hyperadrenocorticism in the ferret. In: Bonagura JD, editor. Kirk's current veterinary therapy XIII, small animal practice. Philadelphia: Saunders; 2000. p. 372–4.

[8] Krogstad AP, Dixon LW. Gross pathology of small mammals. Sem Av Exotic Pet Med 2003; 2:106–21.

[9] Weiss CA, Williams BH, Scott JB, et al. Surgical treatment and long-term outcome of ferrets with bilateral adrenal tumors or adrenal hyperplasia: 56 cases (1994–1997). J Am Vet Med Assoc 1999;215:820–3.

[10] Shoemaker NJ, Schuurmans M, Moorman H, et al. Correlation between age at neutering and age at onset of hyperadrenocorticism in ferrets. J Am Vet Med Assoc 2000;216:195–7.

[11] Wagner RA, Piche CA, Jochle W, et al. Clinical and endocrine responses to treatment with deslorelin acetate implants in ferrets with adrenocortical disease. Am J Vet Res 2005;66: 910–4.

[12] Peterson RA, Kiupel M, Capen CC. Adrenal cortical carcinomas with myxoid differentiation in the domestic ferret (*Mustela putorius furo*). Vet Pathol 2003;40:136–42.

[13] Bielinska M, Kiiveri S, Parviainen H, et al. Gonadectomy-induced adrenocortical neoplasia in the domestic ferret (*Mustela putorius furo*) and laboratory mouse. Vet Pathol 2006;43: 97–117.

[14] Johnson-Delaney CA. Medical therapies for ferret adrenal disease. Sem Av Exotic Pet Med 2004;13(1):3–7.

[15] Ramer JC, Benson KG, Morrisey JK, et al. Effects of melatonin administration on the clinical course of adrenocortical disease in domestic ferrets. J Am Vet Med Assoc 2006;229: 1743–8.

[16] Wagner RA, Bailey EM, Schneider JF, et al. Leuprolide acetate treatment of adrenocortical disease in ferrets. J Am Vet Med Assoc 2001;218:1272–4.

[17] Johnson-Delaney CA, Update of ferret adrenal disease: etiology, diagnosis, and treatment. Proceedings of the Conference of the Association of Avian Veterinarians 2006;69–74.

[18] Peterson RA, Kiupel M, Bielinska M, et al. Transcription factor GATA-4 is a marker of anaplasia in adrenocortical neoplasms of the domestic ferret (*Mustela putorius furo*). Vet Pathol 2004;41:446–9.

[19] Newman SJ, Bergman PJ, Williams B, et al. Characterization of spindle cell component of ferret (*Mustela putorius furo*) adrenal cortical neoplasms - a correlation to clinical parameters and prognosis. Veterinary Comparative Oncology 2004;2:113–24.

[20] Bartlett LW. Ferret soft tissue surgery. Sem Av Exotic Pet Med 2002;11(4):221–30.

[21] Rosenthal KL, Peterson ME. Evaluation of plasma androgen and estrogen concentrations in ferrets with hyperadrenocorticism. J Am Vet Med Assoc 1996;209:1097–102.

[22] Coleman GD, Chavez MA, Williams BH. Cystic prostatic disease associated with adrenocortical lesions in the ferret (*Mustela putorius furo*). Vet Pathol 1998;35:546–9.

[23] Rosenthal KL, Peterson ME, Quesenberry KE, et al. Hyperadrenocorticism associated with adrenocortical tumor or nodular hyperplasia of the adrenal gland in ferrets: 50 cases (1987–1991). J Am Vet Med Assoc 1993;203:271–5.

[24] Besso JG, Tidwell AS, Gliatto JM. Retrospective review of the ultrasonographic features of adrenal lesions in 21 ferrets. Vet Radiol Ultrasound 2000;41:345–52.

[25] Kuijten AM, Shoemaker NJ, Voorhout G. Ultrasonographic visualization of the adrenal glands of healthy ferrets and ferrets with hyperadrenocorticism. J Am Anim Hosp Assoc 2007;43:78–84.

[26] Neuwirth L, Collins B, Calderwood-Mays M, et al. Adrenal ultrasonography correlated with histopathology in ferrets. Vet Radiol Ultrasound 1997;38:69–74.

[27] Schoemaker NJ, Lumeij JT, Rijnberk A. Plasma concentrations of adrenocorticotrophic hormone and a-melanocyte-stimulating hormone in ferrets (*Mustela putorius furo*) with hyperadrenocorticism. Am J Vet Res 2002;63:1395–9.

[28] Schoemaker NJ, Wolfswinkel J, Mol JA, et al. Urinary glucocorticoid excretion in the diagnosis of hyperadrenocorticism in ferrets. Domest Anim Endocrinol 2004;27:13–24.

[29] Ottinger MA, Wu J, Pelican K. Neuroendocrine regulation of reproduction in birds and clinical applications of GnRH analogues in birds and mammals. Sem Av Exotic Pet Med 2002;11(2):71–9.

[30] Plumb DC. Melatonin. In: Veterinary drug handbook. 4th edition. Ames (IA): Iowa State Press; 2002. p. 515–6.

[31] Plumb DC. Mitotane. In: Veterinary drug handbook. 4th edition. Ames (IA): Iowa State Press; 2002. p. 564–6.

ELSEVIER
SAUNDERS

VETERINARY
CLINICS
Exotic Animal Practice

Vet Clin Exot Anim 11 (2008) 139–152

Hormonal Regulation and Calcium Metabolism in the Rabbit

Christine Eckermann-Ross, DVM, CVA[a,b,*]

[a]Avian and Exotic Animal Care, PA, 8711 Fidelity Boulevard, Raleigh, NC 27617, USA
[b]North Carolina State University College of Veterinary Medicine, 4700 Hillsborough Street, Raleigh, NC 27606, USA

Calcium is an important mineral in homeostasis in all vertebrate animals. It is the most abundant mineral in the body, and is the major component of bones and teeth. In addition, calcium is involved in various vital physiologic processes, including blood coagulation, muscle contraction, membrane permeability, nerve conduction, enzyme activity, and hormone release. Calcium balance is achieved by the interaction of various control mechanisms that regulate its absorption and excretion. Parathyroid hormone (PTH), calcitonin, and vitamin D are the primary regulators of calcium homeostasis. Other minerals, including phosphate and magnesium, and other hormones, such as estrogen, testosterone, steroid hormones, and glucagon, also play a role. In most mammals, the interaction of these regulatory mechanisms maintains serum calcium levels within a narrow range. In contrast, rabbits have adapted a unique strategy in which most dietary calcium is absorbed in the intestine, and the excess is excreted in the urine. In this species, calcium levels may vary within a wide range, and in direct proportion to the dietary calcium intake. This unique calcium metabolism has implications for the health and husbandry of the rabbit.

Review of normal calcium metabolism

Approximately 95% of body calcium is found combined with phosphate in the inorganic matrix of bone. One percent is found in the cell cytoplasm sequestered in the plasma membrane and endoplasmic reticulum, and the remaining 4% is found in the plasma [1]. Plasma calcium is present in three

* Avian and Exotic Animal Care, PA, 8711 Fidelity Boulevard, Raleigh, NC 27617.
E-mail address: drdan@avianandexotic.com

forms. Free, or ionized, calcium comprises about 55% of plasma calcium. The remainder is found complexed with anions, such as bicarbonate, citrate, phosphate, and lactate, or is bound to proteins [2]. The protein with the highest calcium-binding affinity is albumin, and plasma albumin levels affect the assessment of total blood calcium concentration. Serum ionized calcium concentrations have been demonstrated to be linearly related to total calcium concentrations [3]. Ionized calcium levels are pH-dependent and are affected by acid-base disorders [4].

Dietary calcium is the only exogenous calcium source, while bone remodeling serves as an endogenous calcium reservoir. In most mammals, dietary calcium is absorbed from the intestine by two processes. Passive diffusion occurs along the calcium concentration gradient between the blood and intestinal lumen. Active transport is a vitamin D–dependent process. Active vitamin D3 stimulates the formation of a calcium-binding protein in the intestinal epithelium that functions at the brush border to transport calcium into the cell cytoplasm [5]. This process is also influenced by intestinal calcium concentrations [6]. The pituitary hormones prolactin and growth hormone enhance, and glucocorticoids inhibit, this active transport [2,7]. Urinary excretion is the principal route of calcium loss from the body. Fecal excretion, sweat, tooth formation, pancreatic and biliary secretions, lactation, and pregnancy or egg formation are also routes of calcium loss or increased metabolic demand for calcium [1,4].

Normal calcium metabolism in the rabbit

Calcium metabolism in the rabbit differs in several respects from that of other mammals. In most species, calcium absorption is closely regulated to balance metabolic needs, and serum calcium concentrations are maintained within a narrow range, typically 1.25 to 1.6 mmol/L (5.0–6.4 mg/dL) [2]. Total serum calcium in the rabbit is 30% to 50% higher than in other mammals, and varies over a wide range, from 3.25 to 3.75 mmol/L (13–15 mg/dL). Ionized serum calcium in the rabbit is approximately 1.71 ± 0.11 mmol/L [8]. In most species, a PTH response is initiated when serum ionized calcium levels fall to 1.2 mmol/L, whereas in the rabbit, a PTH response is triggered at 1.7 mmol/L [3].

The intestinal absorption of calcium in most mammals involves primarily vitamin D3–regulated active transport. In the rabbit, however, passive absorption according to a concentration gradient between the blood and intestinal lumen predominates [6,9]. The amount of calcium absorbed increases in proportion to the amount of calcium in the diet, and is relatively independent of vitamin D [3,8]. When a high-fat diet is fed to rabbits experimentally, the fat chelates the calcium in the gastrointestinal tract, rendering it less available to the rabbit. Although control rabbits excreted 20% of ingested calcium in the feces, rabbits fed high dietary fat excreted 30% in the feces. However, 56% of the ingested calcium was still excreted in the urine, demonstrating an extremely efficient mechanism for intestinal absorption of calcium [10]. In contrast to most mammalian species, which grow only one or two sets of teeth in their lifetime, a rabbit's teeth are constantly erupting at a rate of approximately 2 to 2.4 mm/week [11]. This increased life-long demand for calcium, compared with other mammals, is met by the efficient calcium absorption described earlier. In addition, during normal dental wear, calcium is released from the teeth, swallowed, and reabsorbed from the intestine [4].

In the mammalian nephron, 60% to 65% of filtered calcium is reabsorbed in the proximal tubule, and less than 2% of the filtered load is excreted in the urine. A rise in serum calcium concentration, increased glomerular filtration rate, or decreased tubular reabsorption of calcium will result in increased calciuria [12,13]. In the rabbit, calcium is absorbed in direct proportion to the amount ingested in the diet, rather than in accordance with metabolic need. Urinary calcium excretion increases in parallel to dietary intake [10,14,15]. The fraction of calcium that can be filtered out of the blood is higher than in other mammals, and fractional excretion of calcium in the urine can reach 44.9% [16]. In one study, rabbits excreted about 60% of ingested calcium in the urine, whereas in rats, only 2% of ingested calcium was eliminated by way of this route [10]. When the reabsorptive capacity of the kidney is reached, calcium precipitates as calcium carbonate in the alkaline urine of the rabbit, causing cloudy or sludgy urine. When metabolic demand for calcium is increased by growth, pregnancy, lactation, or metabolic disorders, less calcium is excreted and the urine appears clear [6,17].

Hormonal regulation of calcium metabolism

The main hormonal regulators of calcium homeostasis are PTH, calcitonin, and active vitamin D3 (1,25 $(OH)_2D3$). Other hormones, including estrogen, testosterone, prolactin, growth hormone, glucagon, and gastrin, and corticosteroids and other minerals also play a role in calcium regulation.

Parathyroid hormone

PTH is the principal hormone involved in minute-to-minute fine regulation of blood calcium in mammals. It is secreted by the chief cells of the parathyroid gland in response to decreases in serum ionized calcium or 1,25 $(OH)_2D3$ concentrations [2]. In the kidney, PTH acts on the renal tubules to increase calcium reabsorption and promote phosphorous excretion. By increasing the activity of alpha-hydroxylase in renal tubules, PTH is also a major stimulator of renal 1,25 $(OH)_2D3$ synthesis, which increases duodenal calcium absorption. In bone, PTH stimulates osteoclastic bone resorption, thus increasing the release of calcium and phosphate into the blood. PTH levels have been shown to rise postprandially, stimulating the release of gastrin and digestive hormones, which are postulated to affect serum calcium concentrations [1]. The end result of these actions is a rise in serum calcium concentration, which inhibits further release of PTH by negative feedback. These actions also result in decreased urinary calcium excretion [18,19].

Rabbits exhibit a unique pattern of renal response to PTH. The rabbits' ionized calcium concentration is protected from hyper- and hypocalcemia by rapidly changing PTH and calcitonin secretion. Changes in PTH secretion are seen only at relatively high calcium concentrations, levels that are the physiologic norm for the rabbit. Despite having a high serum calcium concentration, rabbits have readily measurable levels of PTH, which are dramatically reduced by infusion of calcium, implying that the parathyroid gland and PTH actively contribute to calcium homeostasis in this species. The effects noted are qualitatively similar to the effects of PTH in rats, but significant increases in phosphate excretion occur only at very high doses of PTH, and much larger changes in calcium excretion are noted [3,20]. In vitro perfusion studies of the rabbit nephron have demonstrated that PTH increases calcium transport in the cortical segment of the loop of Henle, but not in the medullary segment [21,22], and causes an increase in calcium absorption in the connecting tubule [23,24]. It is the distal nephron segments that play the key role in determining the calcium excretion in the final urine, and this content is regulated by the actions of PTH and calcitonin, and the presence of other minerals, particularly sodium [12,25–28].

Calcitonin

Calcitonin is produced by the C cells of the thyroid gland and released in response to increases in plasma calcium concentration. Release of calcitonin is also enhanced by estradiol, glucagons, and gastrointestinal hormones, including gastrin, cholecystokinin, and secretin. Calcitonin levels increase postprandially, especially after a high-calcium meal. Neonates and pregnant and lactating animals also demonstrate increased calcitonin levels [1,22,29]. Calcitonin decreases PTH-stimulated osteoclastic bone resorption and lowers the cytosolic calcium concentration in bone cells, thus decreasing calcium efflux from the pool of labile bone calcium. The hormone may aid in sequestering calcium and phosphate in bone in a form in which it could be available for fasting needs. Renal tubular reabsorption of calcium and phosphate are decreased by calcitonin. In the gastrointestinal tract, calcitonin causes decreased secretion of gastrin and gastric acid, and causes increased small bowel secretion of sodium, potassium, chloride, and water. No major effect has been shown on the regulation of intestinal calcium absorption [30]. The end result of these actions is a lowering of serum calcium concentration.

Species variability in the role of calcitonin in calcium homeostasis is marked. In the lower vertebrates, calcitonin has a potent hypocalcemic effect, whereas in humans, the effect on plasma calcium concentration is minor, and the hormone is viewed as an "emergency" hormone to prevent the acute development of hypercalcemia [22,29]. In thyroparathyroidectomized rats, calcitonin infusion produced hypocalcemia and reduced urinary calcium excretion [31,32]. Another group demonstrated that a moderate dose of calcitonin caused a reduction in urinary calcium, whereas repeated daily administration resulted in increased calciuria in rats [33]. Still another study demonstrated a hypocalcemic effect, but no effect on urine parameters [34]. When calcitonin is administered by injection to human patients with hypercalcemia, tubular reabsorption of calcium is decreased, resulting in decreased serum calcium concentration and increased urinary excretion of calcium [35,36]. In the lamb, calcitonin increased urinary excretion of calcium, whereas in the dog and rabbit, calcium excretion was unaffected [21].

In vitro studies with isolated rabbit nephrons have demonstrated specific calcitonin receptors in the kidney that are distinct from PTH receptors [37]. The hormone increased net calcium flux in distal portions of the nephrons, resulting in an overall calciuric effect in vitro [23,36,38]. Still, the physiologic effects of calcitonin in the rabbit remain unclear. One group found that intramuscular injections of calcitonin decreased serum calcium concentration [39], whereas another concluded that the concentration did not change [40]. No consistent effect has been demonstrated on urinary excretion of calcium in the rabbit [20,40].

Vitamin D

The precursors of active vitamin D3 come from the diet or are synthesized in the epidermis from 7-dehydrocholesterol. The conversion of 7-dehydrocholesterol is catalyzed by ultraviolet irradiation from sunlight. Dietary precursors are absorbed in the proximal small intestine and modified by hydroxylation in the liver and kidneys. In the kidney, activation of the enzyme 1-alpha-hydroxylase results in the final conversion of 25-hydroycholicalciferol to 1,25 $(OH)_2D3$. Synthesis of active vitamin D3 is stimulated by PTH, and may also be increased by prolactin, estradiol, and growth hormone. Increased serum calcium and vitamin D concentrations will decrease the rate of conversion to active vitamin D3. The main function of vitamin D is to regulate the absorption of enough calcium and phosphorus to ensure adequate concentrations for bone mineralization. In most mammals, vitamin D is the principal regulator of intestinal calcium and phosphorus absorption. The hormone is also necessary for osteoclastic bone resorption and mobilization of calcium from bone, and increases renal tubular reabsorption of calcium and phosphorus [1,22,41,42]. Vitamin D also decreases the formation and secretion of PTH by the parathyroid gland [43].

When rabbits are fed a diet deficient in vitamin D, serum PTH levels rise, but serum calcium levels do not change detectably [44]. Chronically vitamin D–deficient rabbits showed no change in net intestinal absorption of calcium or phosphorus, compared with controls, whereas urinary excretion of both minerals was decreased. These results emphasize the vitamin

D–independent nature of intestinal calcium absorption in the rabbit, and the importance of renal conservation of calcium and phosphorus in vitamin D–deficient rabbits [9]. Vitamin D also plays a role in insulin secretion and glucose tolerance in the rabbit [45], and helps maintain the transplacental calcium gradient in pregnant does [46].

Other hormonal regulators of calcium homeostasis

In humans, estrogen and androgens are known to regulate renal calcium transport. This regulatory effect may partly account for the negative calcium balance that results from deficiency of these hormones [47]. Estrogens also increase intestinal absorption of calcium and elevate total serum calcium concentration, and may influence the conversion to active vitamin D3 [42,48]. Testosterone [49] and progesterone [50] enhance the reabsorption of calcium in the rabbit kidney. Prolactin is known to induce hypercalcemia in chicks, quail, frogs, and humans [42,51]. In rats given intravenous prolactin, serum calcium increased by 4.8% and urinary excretion of calcium by 36% [52]. When neutered rats were fed a lithogenic diet, the incidence of urinary stone formation decreased by 10%, compared with intact animals on the same diet. When testosterone was administered, 80% of the animals developed urolithiasis. The incidence of urinary stones in intact female rats fed the same diet and given testosterone was 10%, and increased to 40% in oophorectomized females. These results suggest that testosterone may have a determinant effect in the formation of urinary stones, and estrogen may have a protective effect [53,54]. It would be interesting to note any similar effects in rabbits, and to determine the effects of gonadectomy on calcium homeostasis in the rabbit. Sex steroids have also been shown to play a role in decreasing the calcium content of atherosclerotic plaques in spayed rabbits fed a high-cholesterol diet [55].

Prostaglandins (PG) of the E series are potent activators of bone resorption. PGE 1 causes increased synthesis of active vitamin D and subsequent hyperabsorption of calcium at the intestinal level. When administered intravenously to rabbits, PGE 1 increased serum calcium concentration [56]. PGE 2 increases osteoclast numbers, leading to increased bone resorption [29].

Exogenous steroid administration and endogenous glucocorticoids have been associated with decreased intestinal calcium absorption and increased renal calcium loss [57]. Adrenal cortical steroids have actions that are antagonistic to vitamin D and PTH, and can affect the responses of plasma calcium, phosphorus, PTH, and calcitonin [58–60]. Administration of dexamethasone to rabbits resulted in calcium retention in the wall of the duodenum [61]. Suckling rabbits treated with methylprednisolone exhibited decreased intestinal calcium absorption and increased renal calcium loss, and developed secondary hyperparathyroidism [62]. Another group found decreased serum $1,25(OH)_2D3$ concentration, decreased bone trabecular volume, and an increased rate of bone turnover in methylprednisolone-treated rabbits [59].

Growth hormone is the principal hormone regulator of growth. It causes increased intestinal calcium absorption in humans, and has been shown to produce hypercalciuria by an unknown mechanism. Growth hormone may also produce hypercalcemia, possibly by stimulating 1,25 $(OH)_2D3$ production [60].

Several digestive and pancreatic hormones also affect mineral homeostasis. Insulin deficiency results in decreased intestinal calcium absorption in association with low levels of vitamin D. Pharmacologic doses of glucagons produce transient hypocalcemia, but the physiologic role of this hormone is not clear [60,63]. The hypocalcemic effect of glucagon may depend on the presence of the thyroid gland in rabbits [64]. Gastrin, secretin, and vasoactive intestinal peptide have been shown to alter extracellular calcium concentrations in animals, but their physiologic role has not been determined [60]. It has been proposed that the association of the digestive enzymes and calcitonin in the postprandial period may affect the hypocalcemic effects of these hormones and may also explain the hypocalcemia seen in some cases of pancreatitis [29,61].

Medical disorders associated with abnormal calcium metabolism

Urolithiasis and "sludgy" urine

The urine of rabbits is normally cloudy in appearance and contains three main types of calcium-containing crystals: calcium carbonate monohydrate, anhydrous calcium carbonate, and ammonium magnesium phosphate [65]. Urolithiasis and "sludgy" urine are common in rabbits, and may result from an exacerbation of normal physiologic calcium excretion [66–68]. When rabbits are fed a high-calcium diet, urinary calcium excretion increases, but urine volume remains constant, increasing the likelihood of crystal aggregation and stone formation [8]. The alkaline pH of rabbit urine also increases the risk of forming insoluble calcium precipitates [69]. Genetic predisposition, dehydration, metabolic disorders, bacterial or parasitic infections, and nutritional imbalances may also be predisposing factors. Temporary obstruction of the kidney in rabbits recovering from hydronephrosis resulted in crystal aggregation and stone formation within a few weeks [70]. This finding suggests that any condition causing urinary stasis (arthritis, *Encephalitozoon cuniculi* infection, spinal trauma or deformity, bacterial infection, lack of exercise, obesity) may also predispose the rabbit to urolithiasis [4].

Dental disease

Dental disease and its sequelae (anorexia, poor grooming, jaw abscesses, nasolacrimal duct obstruction, and epiphora) are among the most common medical problems in pet rabbits. Predisposing factors include abnormal wear, disease of the temporomandibular joint, ageing, decreased dietary

fiber, genetic predisposition, and metabolic bone disease. Rabbits with corticosteroid-induced osteoporosis showed three to four times greater orthodontic tooth movement and less tooth stability, compared with controls
[71]. In rabbits with acquired dental disease, serum calcium levels are decreased and PTH levels are increased, compared with normal [72]. In a study
of 40 rabbits with acquired dental disease, poor tooth and bone quality was
the most important etiologic factor, with an apparent underlying osteodystrophy and failure of calcification of the skull and teeth [73]. Nutritional investigation of this osteodystrophic condition suggests that selective feeding
behavior of pet rabbits may result in an unbalanced ratio of calcium and
phosphorus, leading to nutritional osteodystrophy [74]. Another study
found that rabbits with dental disease that were kept in hutches had increased PTH and decreased calcium levels, compared with free-range rabbits
allowed to forage naturally [72]. This finding also supports the assertion that
selective feeding and inadequate calcium intake may be predisposing factors
in acquired dental disease in rabbits.

Chronic renal failure

Chronic renal failure has been reported in pet rabbits and is associated
with polyuria and polydipsia, decreased activity level, anorexia, and weight
loss. In rabbits with renal failure induced by partial nephrectomy, serum calcium levels are increased, whereas serum PTH is markedly decreased. If
these same rabbits are fed a calcium-deficient diet, serum calcium is
decreased and PTH is increased, and secondary hyperparathyroidism and
adynamic bone disease may result [75]. Additionally, the increased PTH
in the blood of uremic rabbits increases the influx of calcium into red blood
cells, increasing their osmotic fragility. Thus, anemia in rabbits with renal
failure may be the result of the role of PTH in increasing red blood cell
fragility [76]. When intestinal calcium absorption continues, but renal excretion of calcium is impaired, soft tissue mineralization may result [4].

Hypercalcemia and hypocalcemia

Hypercalcemia has been reported in rabbits, and may result from primary
or secondary hyperparathyroidism, hypervitaminosis D, osteolytic bone tumors or septic osteomyelitis, granulomatous disease, severe hypothermia, or
renal disease. One rabbit with hypercalcemia (serum calcium concentration
of 19.8 mg/dL) exhibited anorexia, weight loss, diarrhea, renal calcification,
and other renal abnormalities [77]. Spontaneous aortic arteriosclerosis has
been reported in hypercalcemic rabbits [78] and in rabbits fed a diet high
in calcium and vitamin D [8,79,80]. Hypercalcemia commonly depressed
renal function and urinary concentrating capacity [81]. Another report
describes hypercalcemia in a rabbit with thymoma, suggesting hypercalcemia as a paraneoplastic syndrome in this species [82].

When rabbits are fed a diet deficient in calcium, hypocalcemia may result. Rabbits consuming a low-calcium and high-phosphorous diet developed increased serum PTH, hypocalcemia, hyperphosphatemia, and hypovitaminosis D, rapidly resulting in nutritional secondary hyperparathyroidism [83] and decreased bone mass [84,85]. When alveolar bone is lost, the bone of the mandible may be most affected, and acquired dental disease may be the end result [4]. Dietary calcium restriction during growth reduces peak bone mass at skeletal maturity [86]. Hypocalcemia often occurs in the periparturient period, and has been reported in does with pregnancy toxemia. Affected rabbits may exhibit weakness, depression, ataxia, anorexia, convulsion, and coma. Urinary calcium excretion is decreased and the urine becomes clear and acidic [87].

Vitamin D deficiency and toxicosis

Rabbits have a lower requirement for vitamin D than other mammals, and as little as a five-times increase over normal dietary levels (> 3000 mg/kg) may result in intoxication [88]. Vitamin D toxicosis is characterized by anorexia, weight loss and weakness, diarrhea, polydipsia, paralysis, and soft tissue calcification [89]. Independent of the calcium intake, increasing vitamin D levels in the diet of rabbits increases calcium content in aortic tissue [8].

Vitamin D deficiency presents with anemia, predisposition to infection, impaired immune system function, and depression of inflammatory responses [41]. In rabbits, chronic feeding of a vitamin D–deficient diet resulted in inadequate skeletal mineralization and signs of osteomalacia. These symptoms appeared to be caused by hypophosphatemia, rather than hypocalcemia [44].

Dietary considerations

The unusual calcium metabolism of rabbits makes it essential to maintain a diet that is well balanced, with appropriate calcium concentration, calcium-to-phosphorus ratio, and vitamin D content. If too little calcium is consumed, secondary hyperparathyroidism and bone resorption may result, whereas if too much calcium is present, the risk of urolithiasis is increased [74]. A dietary calcium level of 0.22% supports normal growth, but 0.35% to 0.4% calcium is required for optimal bone calcification and growth rates in young rabbits [90,91]. Prevention of soft tissue mineralization requires less than 25 µg (1000 IU) cholecalciferol per kilogram of food [69]. The pet rabbit's diet should be chosen carefully to prevent selective feeding. If the rabbit rejects pellets and whole grain, calcium intake may be insufficient [74]. Most commercial rabbit feeds contain calcium from alfalfa hay and calcium carbonate, which are very absorbable. Although many vegetables are high in calcium, they often contain calcium oxalate, which is not metabolized by rabbits, and thus, cannot contribute to urine sludge [6,11]. The ideal diet for pet rabbits should contain 15% to 16% fiber, 12% to 13% protein, 1% to 3% fat, 0.6% to 1.0% calcium, should have a calcium-to-phosphorus ratio of 1:1 to 2:1, and should have fewer than 1000 IU/kg vitamin D [89,92]. A diet comprising grass hay versus legume hay, a small portion of commercial pellets composed of timothy hay, fresh vegetables, and fresh drinking water has been recommended [6,8,74].

Acknowledgments

The author thanks Dr. Daniel H. Johnson and Dr. Edgar H. Eckermann for their critical review of this article.

References

[1] Ruckebusch Y, Phaneuf LP, Dunlop R. Physiology of small and large animals. Philadelphia: B.C. Decker, Inc; 1991. p. 521–6.

[2] Rosol TJ, Capen CC. Calcium-regulating hormones and diseases of abnormal mineral (calcium, phosphorous, magnesium) metabolism. In: Kaneko JJ, Harvey JW, Bruss ML, editors. Clinical biochemistry of domestic animals. 5th edition. San Diego (CA): Academic Press; 1997. p. 619–702.

[3] Warren HB, Lausen NC, Segre GV, et al. Regulation of calciotropic hormones in vivo in the New Zealand white rabbit. Endocrinology 1989;125(5):2683–90.

[4] Harcourt-Brown MF. Calcium metabolism in rabbits. Exotic DVM Magazine 2005;6(2): 11–4.

[5] Reece WO. Functional anatomy and physiology of domestic animals. 3rd edition. Philadelphia: Lippincott, Williams & Wilkins; 2005. p. 293, 465.

[6] Redrobe S. Calcium metabolism in rabbits. Seminars in avian and exotic pet medicine 2002; 11(2):94–101.

[7] Levine BS, Walling MW, Coburn JW. Intestinal absorption of calcium; its assessment, normal physiology, and alterations in various disease states. In: Bronner F, Coburn JW, editors. Disorders of mineral metabolism, vol. 2, calcium physiology. New York: Academic Press; 1982. p. 104–88.

[8] Kamphues J, Carstensen D, Schroeder D, et al. Effects of increasing calcium and vitamin D supply on calcium metabolism of rabbits. J Anim Physiol Anim Nutr 1986;56: 191–208.

[9] Bourdeau JE, Schwer-Dymerski DA, Stern PH, et al. Calcium and phosphorus metabolism in chronically vitamin D deficient laboratory rabbits. Miner Electrolyte Metab 1986;12: 176–85.

[10] Cheeke PR, Amberg JW. Comparative calcium excretion by rats and rabbits. J Anim Sci 1973;37(2):450–4.

[11] Shadle AR. The attrition and extrusive growth of the four major incisor teeth of domestic rabbits. Journal of Mammology 1936;17:15–21.

[12] Shareghi GR, Stoner LC. Calcium transport across segments of the rabbit distal nephron in vitro. Am J Physiol 1978;235(4):F367–75.

[13] Massry SG. Renal handling of calcium. In: Bronner F, Coburn JW, editors. Disorders of mineral metabolism, vol. 2, calcium physiology. New York: Academic Press; 1982. p. 189–235.

[14] Kennedy A. The urinary excretion of calcium by normal rabbits. J Comp Pathol 1965;75: 69–74.

[15] Whiting SJ, Quamme GA. Effects of dietary calcium on renal calcium, magnesium and phosphate excretion by the rabbit. Miner Electrolyte Metab 1984;10:217–21.

[16] Buss SL, Bourdeau JE. Calcium balance in laboratory rabbits. Miner Electrolyte Metab 1984;10:127–32.

[17] Harcourt-Brown F. Textbook of rabbit medicine. Oxford (UK): Butterworth Heineman; 2002. p. 19–51, 185–92, 339.

[18] Berndt T, Marchand T, Sell T, et al. The effects of parathyroid hormone (PTH) and calcitonin (CT) on electrolyte and cyclic AMP (cAMP) excretion in the rabbit. Fed Proc 1978;37(3): 728.

[19] Habener JF, Rosenblatt M, Potts JT. Parathyroid hormone: biochemical aspects of biosynthesis, secretion, action and metabolism. Physiol Rev 1984;64(3):985–1053.

[20] Berndt TJ, Knox FG. Effects of parathyroid hormone and calcitonin on electrolyte excretion in the rabbit. Kidney Int 1980;17:473–8.

[21] Suki WN, Rouse D. Hormonal regulation of calcium transport in thick ascending limb renal tubules. Am J Physiol 1981;241(Renal fluid electrolyte Physiol 10):F171–4.

[22] Rocha AS, Magaldi JB, Kokko JP. Calcium and phosphate transport in isolated segments of rabbit Henle's loop. J Clin Invest 1977;59:975–83.

[23] Shimzu T, Yoshitomi K, Nakamura M, et al. Effects of PTH, calcitonin and cAMP on calcium transport in rabbit distal nephron segments. Am J Physiol 1990;259(Renal fluid electrolyte Physiol 28):F408–14.

[24] Imai M. Effects of parathyroid hormone and N6 O2-dibutyryl cyclic AMP on Ca2+ transport across the rabbit distal nephron segments perfused in vitro. Pflugers Arch 1981;390: 145–51.

[25] Brunette MG, Mailloux J, Lajeunesse D. Calcium transport through the luminal membrane of the distal tubule. I. Interrelationship with sodium. Kidney Int 1992;41:281–8.

[26] Lajeunesse D, Bouhtiauy I, Brunette MG. Parathyroid hormone and hydrochlorothiazide increase calcium transport by the luminal membrane of rabbit distal nephron segments through different pathways. Endocrinology 1994;134(1):35–41.

[27] Morel F. Site of hormone action in the mammalian nephron. Am J Physiol 1981;240(Renal Fluid Electrolyte Physiol):F159–64.

[28] Chabardes D, Imbert M, Clique A, et al. PTH sensitive adenyl cyclase activity in different segments on the rabbit nephron. Pflugers Arch 1975;354:229–39.

[29] Talmage RV, Cooper CW, Toverud SU. The physiologic significance of calcitonin. Bone and Mineral Research 1983;1:74–143.

[30] Austin LA, Heath H. Calcitonin physiology and pathophysiology. N Engl J Med 1981; 304(5):269–76.

[31] Kisloff B, Moore EW. Effects of intravenous calcitonin on water, electrolyte and calcium movement across in vivo rabbit jejunum and ileum. Gastroenterology 1977;72(3):462–8.

[32] Quamme GA. Effect of calcitonin on calcium and magnesium transport in rat nephron. Am J Physiol 1980;238(Endocrinol metab 1):E573–5.

[33] Talmage RV, Grubb SA. The influence of endogenous or exogenous calcitonin on daily urinary calcium excretion. Endocrinology 1977;101:1351–7.

[34] Aldred JP, Kleszynski RR, Bostian JW. Effects of acute administration of porcine and salmon calcitonin on urine electrolyte excretion in rats. Proc Soc Exp Biol Med 1970;134: 1175–9.

[35] Cochran M, Peacock M, Sachs G, et al. Renal effects of calcitonin. Br Med J 1970;1:135–7.

[36] Zuo Q, Claveau D, Hilal G, et al. Effect of calcitonin on calcium transport by the luminal and basolateral membranes of the rabbit nephron. Kidney Int 1997;51:1991–9.

[37] Aurbach GD, Heath DA. Parathyroid hormone and calcitonin regulation of renal function. Kidney Int 1974;6:331–45.

[38] Chabardes D, Imbert-Teboul M, Montegut M, et al. Distribution of calcitonin-sensitive adenylate cyclase activity along the rabbit kidney tubule. Proc Natl Acad Sci U S A 1976; 73(10):3608–12.

[39] Luplescu A. Effect of synthetic salmon calcitonin on glucose, blood urea nitrogen and serum electrolytes in rabbits. J Pharmacol Exp Ther 1974;188(2):318–23.

[40] Salako LA, Smith AJ, Smith RN. The effects of porcine calcitonin on renal function in the rabbit. J Endocrinol 1971;50:485–91.

[41] Bell NH. Vitmain D—endocrine system. J Clin Invest 1985;76:1–6.

[42] Fraser DR. Regulation of the metabolism of vitamin D. Physiol Rev 1980;60(2):551–613.

[43] Sherwood LM, Russell J. The role of 1, 25-$(OH)_2$D3 in regulating parathyroid gland function. Proc Soc Exp Biol Med 1989;191:233–7.

[44] Brommage R, Miller SC, Langman CB, et al. The effects of chronic vitamin D deficiency on the skeleton in the adult rabbit. Bone 1988;9:131–9.

[45] Nyomba BL, Bouillon R, DeMoor P. Influence of vitamin D status on insulin secretion and glucose tolerance in the rabbit. Endocrinology 1984;115:191–7.

[46] Kubota M, Ohno J, Shiina Y, et al. Vitamin D metabolism in pregnant rabbits: differences between the maternal and fetal response to administration of large amounts of vitamin D3. Endocrinology 1982;110:1950–6.

[47] Dick IM, Liu J, Glendenning P, et al. Estrogen and androgen regulation of plasma membrane calcium pump activity in immortalized distal tubule kidney cells. Mol Cell Endocrinol 2003;212:11–8.

[48] Burnette MG, Leclerc M. Effect of estrogen on calcium and sodium transport by the nephron luminal membranes. J Endocrinol 2001;170:441–50.

[49] Couchourel D, Leclerc M, Filep J, et al. Testosterone enhances calcium reabsorption by the kidney. Mol Cell Endocrinol 2004;222:71–81.

[50] Burnette MG, Leclerc M. Renal action of progesterone: effect on calcium reabsorption. Mol Cell Endocrinol 2002;194:183–90.

[51] Spanos E, Pike JW, Haussler MB, et al. Circulating 1-alpha-25-dihydroxy vitamin D in the chicken; enhancement by injection of prolactin during egg laying. Life Sci 1976;19:1751–6.

[52] Mahajan KK, Robinson CJ, Horrobin DF. Prolactin and hypercalcemia. Lancet 1974;303(7868):1237–8.

[53] Lee YH, Huang WC, Huang JK, et al. Testosterone enhances whereas estrogen inhibits calcium oxalate stone formation in ethylene glycol treated rats. J Urol 1996;156:502–5.

[54] Lee Y, Huang W, chiang H, et al. Determinant role of testosterone in the pathogenesis of urolithiasis in rats. J Urol 1992;147:1134–8.

[55] Aldrighi JM, Lanz JR, Mansur TLR, et al. Effect of sexual steroids on the calcium content of atherosclerotic plaque of oophorectomized rabbits. Braz J Med Biol Res 2005;38:705–11.

[56] Velasquez-Forero F, Garcia P, Triffitt JT, et al. Prostaglandin E1 increases in vivo and in vitro calcitriol biosynthesis in rabbits. Prostaglandins Leukot Essent Fatty Acids 2006;75:107–15.

[57] Kimberg DV, Baerg RD, Geodron E, et al. Effect of cortisone treatment on the active transport of calcium by the small intestine. N Engl J Med 1969;280:1396–405.

[58] Kimberg DV. Effects of vitamin D and steroid hormones on the active transport of calcium by the intestine. N Engl J Med 1969;280(25):1396–405.

[59] Rude RK, Singer FR. Hormonal modifiers of mineral metabolism other than parathyroid hormone, vitamin D, and calcitonin. In: Bronner F, Coburn JW, editors. Disorders of mineral metabolism, vol. 2, calcium physiology. New York: Academic Press; 1982. p. 482–556.

[60] Collette C, Monnier L, Baldet T, et al. Evidence for alterations of vitamin D metabolism in methylprednisolone-treated rabbits. Horm Metab Res 1983;15:249–53.

[61] Eiler H, Lyke A. Retention of calcium in intestinal wall of the rabbit by treatment with a glucocorticoid. Am J Physiol 1983;245(Endocrinol Metab 8):E143–7.

[62] Borowitz SM, Granrud GS. Glucocorticoids inhibit intestinal phosphate absorption in developing rabbits. J Nutr 1992;122:1273–9.

[63] Paloyan E, Paloyan D, Harper PV. Glucagon-induced hypocalcemia. Metabolism 1967;16(1):35–9.

[64] Pickleman JR, Ernst K, Brown S, et al. Glucagon-induced hypocalcemia: effect of the thyroid gland. Surg Forum 1969;20:85–7.

[65] Flatt RE, Carpenter AB. Identification of crystalline material in urine of rabbits. Am J Vet Res 1971;32(4):655–8.

[66] Whary MT, Peper RL. Calcium carbonate urolithiasis in a rabbit. Lab Anim Sci 1994;44(5): 534–6.

[67] Hoefer HL. Urolithiasis in rabbits and guinea pigs. In: Proceedings of the North American Veterinary Conference. Orlando (FL): 2006. p. 1735–6.

[68] Capello V. Diagnosis and treatment of urolithiasis in pet rabbits. Exotic DVM Magazine 2005;6(2):15–22.

[69] Kamphues J. Calcium metabolism of rabbits as an etiological factor for urolithiasis. J Nutr 1991;121:S95–6.

[70] Itatani H, Yoshioka T, Namiki M, et al. Experimental model of calcium-containing renal stone formation in a rabbit. Investig Urol 1979;17(3):234–40.

[71] Ashcraft MB, Southard KA, Tolley EA. The effect of corticosteroid-induced osteoporosis on orthodontic tooth movement. Am J Orthod Dentofacial Orthop 1992;102:310–9.

[72] Harcourt-Brown FM, Baker SJ. Parathyroid hormone, haematological and biochemical parameters in relation to dental disease and husbandry in rabbits. J Small Anim Pract 2001;42: 130–6.

[73] Harcourt-Brown FM. A review of clinical conditions in pet rabbits associated with their teeth. Vet Rec 1995;137:341–6.

[74] Harcourt-Brown FM. Calcium deficiency, diet and dental disease in pet rabbits. Vet Rec 1996;139:567–71.

[75] Bas S, Bas A, Estepa JC, et al. Parathyroid gland function in the uremic rabbit. Domest Anim Endocrinol 2004;26:99–110.

[76] Bogin E, Malachi Z, Djaldeti M, et al. Effect of parathyroid hormone on the fragility and enzyme activities of red blood cells from young and mature rabbits. J Clin Chem Clin Biochem 1987;25:77–82.

[77] Garibaldi BA, Pecquet Goad ME. Hypercalcemia with secondary nephrolithiasis in a rabbit. Lab Anim Sci 1988;38(3):331–3.

[78] Shell LG, Saunders G. Arteriosclerosis in a rabbit. J Am Vet Med Assoc 1989;194(5):679–80.

[79] Zimmerman JE, Guddens WT, DiGiaborno RF, et al. Soft tissue mineralization in rabbits fed a diet containing excess vitamin D. Lab Anim Sci 1990;40(2):212–5.

[80] Quimby F, Foote R, Profit-Olstad M, et al. Hypercalcemia, hypercalcitoninism and arterial calcification in rabbits fed a diet containing excessive vitamin D and calcium. Lab Anim Sci 1982;32:415.

[81] Henneman PH. Effects of high calcium intakes on renal function. Fed Proc 1959;18:1093–6.

[82] Vernau KM, Grahn BH, Clarke-Scott HA, et al. Thymoma in a geriatric rabbit with hypercalcemia and periodic exophthalmos. J Am Vet Med Assoc 1995;206(6):820–2.

[83] Bas S, Bas A, Lopez I, et al. Nutritional secondary hyperparathyroidism in rabbits. Domest Anim Endocrinol 2005;28:380–90.

[84] Mehrotra M, Gupta SK, Kumar K, et al. Calcium deficiency-induced secondary hyperparathyroidism and osteopenia are rapidly reversible with calcium supplementation in growing rabbit pups. Br J Nutr 2006;95:582–90.

[85] Norris SA, Pettifor JM, Gray DA, et al. Calcium metabolism and bone mass in female rabbits during skeletal maturation: effects of dietary calcium intake. Bone 2001;29(1):62–9.

[86] Gilsanz V, Roe TF, Antunes J, et al. Effect of dietary calcium on bone density in growing rabbits. Am J Physiol 1991;260(Endocrinol Metab 23):E471–6.

[87] Pare JA, Paul-Murphy J. Disorders of reproductive and urinary systems. In: Quesenbery KE, Carpenter JW, editors. Ferrets, rabbits and rodents: clinical medicine and surgery. 2nd edition. Philadelphia: WB Saunders; 2003. p. 183–93.

[88] Fisher PG. Exotic mammal renal disease: causes and clinical presentation. Vet Clin North Am Exot Anim Pract 2001;9(1):33–67.

[89] Cheeke PR. Rabbit feeding and nutrition. Orlando (FL): Academic Press; 1987. p. 106–11, 144–5, 336.

[90] Chapin RE, Smith SE. The calcium tolerance of growing and reproducing rabbits. Cornell Vet 1967;57:480–91.

[91] Chapin RE, Smith SE. Calcium requirement of growing rabbits. J Anim Sci 1967;26:67–71.

[92] Lowe JA. Pet rabbit feeding and nutrition. In: Blas C, Wiseman J, editors. The nutrition of the rabbit. Cambridge (MA): CABI Publishing; 1998. p. 304–31.

VETERINARY
CLINICS
Exotic Animal Practice

Vet Clin Exot Anim 11 (2008) 153–162

Endocrine Diseases of Rodents

Bobby R. Collins, DVM, MS, DACLAM

Division of Animal Resources, Virginia Commonwealth University,
1101 East Marshall Street, Richmond, VA 23298-0630, USA

The biomedical research community has seized on the propensity of some rodents to develop endocrine diseases in the laboratory environment to use animals as spontaneously occurring models of human disease. The development of the transgenic mouse technology has allowed scientist to develop "designer mice" with added (knock-ins) or deleted (knock-outs) genetic material that allows them to study each alteration that leads to endocrine disease [1]. Although this technology is making a significant contribution to our understanding of endocrine diseases in humans and animals, only the spontaneously occurring disease models are discussed in this article.

Guinea pig (*Cavia porcellus*)

Guinea pigs are one of the most common rodents kept as pets. The diagnosis of endocrine diseases in the guinea pig is rare.

Anatomy

The gross anatomy and the anatomic location of the endocrine organs are typical of a mammal. A detailed description of the gross anatomy of the endocrine glands is available [2–4].

Alopecia of pregnancy and lactation

Females in the later stages of pregnancy or during lactation frequently present with a bilateral alopecia over the lumbosacral or flank area. Nutrition, genetics, and fluctuating hormones have been suggested as factors in the cause of the alopecia [5]. Regrowth of normal hair generally occurs with the cessation of pregnancy and lactation or with ovariohysterectomy.

E-mail address: brcollins@vcu.edu

Ovarian cysts

Ovarian cysts are probably the most common form of endocrine disease that the clinician encounters in the guinea pig. Cystic rete ovary has been diagnosed at necropsy in 76% of guinea pigs between 1.5 and 5 years of age [6]. The 2- to 4-year-old females are most often affected. The cysts can range from 0.5 to 7 cm in diameter, and they tend to increase in size over time. Cysts may be single or multilocular. Both ovaries are frequently involved.

The affected females present with abdominal distention and occasional anorexia, fatigue, and depression, presumably associated with the discomfort attributable to the distention. Breeding sows may have a history of declining fertility after reaching 15 months of age. If the cysts are functional (ie, cause an increase in serum estrogen or progesterone) [7] a bilaterally symmetric, nonpruritic alopecia may be observed in the flank and lumbosacral area.

A confirmed diagnosis of an ovarian cyst can be established by ultrasonography. Examination of the entire reproductive tract is warranted because of the frequent association of leiomyomas, cystic endometrial hyperplasia, and endometritis with the presence of cystic rete ovary. The treatment of this condition is ovariohysterectomy. In the absence of other clinical conditions, the guinea pigs usually make a full recovery. There may be some permanent hair loss associated with the preexisting alopecia, however.

Diabetes mellitus

Spontaneously occurring diabetic mellitus has been reported as a colony-wide problem. Some animals developed chronic weight loss, polydipsia, polyuria, and diabetic cataracts in a biomedical research facility [8]. Glucosuria (>250 mg/100 mL of urine) and an abnormal oral glucose tolerance test were evident by 6 months of age. The fasting blood sugar levels were variable, even in constantly glucosuric animals, and the values were not significantly different from normal animals. Ketonuria was not always present. When it was, the condition was mild, transitory, and not correlated with the severity of the disease. Researchers reported a subclinical form with only minimal clinical and pathologic changes. Most of the guinea pigs did not require treatment, however, and spontaneous remission (ie, no longer glucosuric) seemed to be common [9].

A single case of diabetes has been observed in a pet guinea pig [10]. A female presented with clinical signs of dysuria attributable to cystitis. Once the diagnosis of diabetes mellitus was established, the clinician placed the animal on NPH insulin and received a favorable response. Dietary manipulations are an important part of the treatment of the diabetic patient. Because spontaneous cures may occur, low-fat, high-fiber diets have been recommended to facilitate this transition and as a means of prevention [11,12].

Neoplasia

Spontaneous neoplasms in the guinea pig are rare, and endocrine tumors are the rarest of all. When neoplasia occurs, almost all of the affected animals are older than 3 years of age [13].

An antitumor factor (probably asparaginase) has been demonstrated in the sera of normal guinea pigs [14]. Guinea pigs also posses Kurloff cells (Foa-Kurloff Cells), a subset of a lymphoid cells that are homologs to natural kill (NK) cells in other mammalian species [15]. NK cells have been shown to be cytotoxic to lymphoblast cells in guinea pigs that have guinea pig leukemia [16].

Clinically, when neoplasia is observed, it is usually benign. Almost all of the reported endocrine tumors were observed at necropsy. There have been no reports of parathyroid tumors or pituitary tumors, and only a single report of a pancreatic islet cell adenoma has been made. The remainder of the reported neoplasms involved the thyroid gland and the adrenal gland. Although carcinomas have been reported for both glands, most of the tumors are benign. The treatment for a clinical diagnosis of neoplasia is surgical excision.

The procedures for adrenalectomy [17,18] and thyroidectomy [19] have been described. Guinea pigs recover thyroid activity because of the presence of thyroid rests in the vicinity of the normal anatomic location of the thyroid gland [20]. Caution must be exercised during thyroidectomy to avoid injury to the recurrent laryngeal nerves. Damage to the laryngeal nerves results in permanent alteration in the guinea pigs vocalizations because of paralysis of the laryngeal muscles [21].

Fatty ingrowths of the pancreas

Age-related changes are associated with histologic appearance of the pancreas [22]. Fatty deposits become more prominent in the exocrine pancreas and the islets. The exocrine portion of the pancreas decreases and the portion of islet tissue increases. The fatty infiltration does not seem to cause any physiologic impairment.

Rat (*Rattus rattus*)

The rat is probably the best-described animal species in the world because of its frequent choice as an animal for biomedical research. The extensive body of literature that has been compiled regarding the effects of nutrition on the incidence of diseases and longevity requires our focused attention. Commercial diets for rats and other animal species are readily available, but these diets are developed to promote rapid growth and reproduction characteristic of the early development phase of life. Diets that promote the decreased incidence of disease and increased longevity are absent or limited in their numbers and availability. Rodent studies have illustrated on numerous occasions that reducing calorie intake, protein, and fat reduces the incidence of disease and extends the life of the animals [23].

The steps to apply this information to the animals under our clinical supervision are as follows:

> Survey the biologic literature and become familiar with the diets that each animal species consumes in the wild.
>
> Become knowledgeable about the variety of commercial diets that are available to support each species.
>
> Try to approximate the natural diet by providing a mixture of commercial diets, seeds, fruits, vegetables, grasses, hays, and so forth.
>
> Limit the ad lib exposure to the most concentrated forms of food. (ie, the commercial diets). The exposure to these dietary items can be limited to several hours per day or alternate-day feeding during the week.

The above steps represent a conscious attempt to manage the animal's diet to prevent or reduce the development of obesity, diabetes, neoplasia, renal disease, and liver disease that are so common among rodents in the captive environment. To ensure the likelihood of success, the practitioner and the pet owner must work diligently to manage the diet of the animals under their care at all stages of life. A successful outcome avoids the endocrine disease that causes morbidity and mortality and results in extended longevity for the animals.

Anatomy

The gross anatomy and the anatomic location of the endocrine glands of the rat are typical of most mammals. The pancreas is diffuse and extends from the end of the duodenal loop to the gastrosplenic omentum. The anatomy is discussed in detail elsewhere [24].

Neoplasia

Spontaneous endocrine gland tumors occur at a relatively high frequency in rats. The frequency of individual endocrine gland involvement is highly variable, however.

The chromophobe adenoma is the most common endocrine tumor that the practitioner encounters in clinical practice. The tumor incidence increases with age, and the incidence is higher in females. High-caloric diets and high-protein diets fed ad lib can increase the incidence of tumors dramatically. Grossly, the tumors may have prominent hemorrhagic areas and the tumors can reach 0.5 cm or more in size. The tumors can compress adjacent to the brain tissue giving rise to clinical signs of lethargy, anorexia, and clinically apparent neurologic abnormalities, such as weakness and seizures. There is no effective treatment of pituitary tumors in the rat, and euthanasia is appropriate. Prevention in the form of dietary management early in life should be a goal for the clinician and the pet owner.

Thyroid gland tumors are common in necropsies of large rodent colonies, but the rats rarely exhibit clinical signs. Although the tumors are usually benign, malignant tumors do occur. Parathyroid gland tumors are extremely rare in rats, and only adenomas have been identified.

Adrenal gland tumors occur frequently in rats. Most cortical tumors are adenomas, although adenocarcinomas with metastases have been described. Tumors of the adrenal medulla are mainly pheochromocytoma tumors. Occasionally these tumors invade the surrounding vessel and become metastatic.

Pancreatic tumors are rare in rats. When tumors are present, benign tumors of the islet cells occur at a higher frequency than exocrine tumors. Carcinomas with metastases have been reported.

If tumors of the pancreas, adrenal gland, thyroid, or parathyroid glands are diagnosed by ultrasound, MRI, or exploratory surgery, excision is possible. The odds are that most of the tumors are benign. Debulking of localized tumor masses may also extend the animal's life.

Diabetes mellitus

Several rat models of spontaneously occurring diabetes mellitus have been recognized and developed in the biomedical research environment. Although the occurrence of diabetes mellitus in pet rats is rare, the laboratory manipulations of these mutations are worthy of mention for their preventive value.

The laboratory models are characteristics of maturity-onset diabetes occurring later in life in association with obesity. This metabolic state is marked by moderate hyperinsulinemia and insulin resistance, which contribute to the development of obesity. These diabetic states have multifactorial genetic mutations that exhibit different metabolic mechanisms giving rise to diabetes. It is highly unlikely that the disturbance in a single metabolic pathway gives rise to the diabetic state. Two of these models are as follows:

The Fatty (fa) Rat. This syndrome is caused by an autosomal recessive gene that results in marked obesity but few symptoms of diabetes [25]. Obesity is recognizable at 4 to 5 weeks of age by the large subcutaneous and intraperitoneal fat deposits. The females are infertile, and all animals are hyperphagic and hyperinsulinemic and exhibit insulin resistance. The islet cells undergo hypertrophy and hyperplasia (hence the hyperinsulinemia), but hyperglycemia does not occur.

"BB" Wistar Rat. This diabetic model develops as an insulitis of varying degrees [26]. The diabetes develops between 6 and 12 weeks. The severity of the disease varies with the intensity of the insulitis and the selective destruction of beta cells. The acute onset presentation can result in hyperglycemia, ketosis, and death in a matter of hours. For the more subtle form the only abnormality is glucose intolerance associated with a lesser degree of insulitis and abnormalities of insulin secretion. The more subtle form is more compatible with providing answers to questions about the origins of diabetes because of its more protracted course.

The management of clinical diabetes in all species is a challenge, especially in small mammals. Because hyperglycemia and glucosuria are not constant features of diabetes in rodents, they are even more difficult to manage. Prevention of the disease by a lifetime of dietary management is the wisest course of action.

The mouse (*Mus musculus*)

The mouse has proved to be the most valuable (and most common) research animal available, primarily because of the development of the breeding techniques and the technology to manipulate the mouse genome to produce transgenic animals [1]. Aside from their value as a research animal, they make wonderful, responsive pets for those individuals who love mice.

As previously described for the rat, the incidence of disease and the longevity can be significantly modified by diet. Low-fat, low-protein diets and the decreased caloric density of the diets tend to reduce the incidence of neoplasia, kidney disease, and liver disease, and such diets tend to lengthen the life of the mouse [27,28].

Anatomy

The gross anatomy and the anatomic location of the endocrine glands are similar to the rat. The gross anatomy is described elsewhere [29].

Diabetes-obesity syndromes

Diabetes is rarely diagnosed in pet mice presented to the clinician. There are many mouse models of maturity-onset diabetes, however, with hyperphagia, obesity, and hyperinsulinemia serving as constant features of the syndrome [28].

The genome of each strain of mouse has been manipulated to allow the scientist to study the various genetic and biochemical pathways that lead to the development of diabetes in a mouse model. Among the various models are the Obese (ob) mouse, the Diabetes (db) mouse, the Fat (fat) mouse, the Tubby (tub) mouse, the New Zealand Obese (NZO) mouse, and the KK mouse. Although these animals are not in the pet trade, they are representative of the biologic possibility that diabetes may be seen by a clinician.

Neoplasia

Endocrine tumors are rare in most strains of mice [30]. As is the case with most rodent neoplasms, the incidence is strain- and sex-dependent, and they usually occur after 18 months of age. Benign tumors are more common then malignant tumors. Although endocrine tumors of mice are exploited in the laboratory for various purposes, mice are not likely to present to a practitioner for diagnosis and treatment.

Syrian hamster (*Mesocricetis auratus*)

The major endocrine diseases of the Syrian hamster are related to the high incidence of spontaneously occurring endocrine neoplasms as the animals increase in age.

Anatomy

The gross anatomy of the hamster has been described [31,32]. Special note should be taken of the difference in the size of the adrenal gland between the sexes. The adrenal gland of the adult male is two to three times larger that the adult female because of enlargement of the zona reticularis. This observation is important if ultrasound or other imaging studies are performed on a hamster.

The anatomic location of the endocrine glands is typical of other rodents.

Neoplasia

The incidence of naturally occurring tumors in the golden hamster is significant [33]. The incidence of neoplasia seems to increase dramatically in both sexes after the first year of life. Tumors of the adrenal cortex and thyroid gland are among the most common neoplasms observed in the hamster.

The vast majority of the tumors recorded for hamsters are nonmalignant. Few tumors have been observed in the pancreas, pituitary gland, or parathyroid gland.

The older hamster exhibits a high incidence of spontaneous lesions in the adrenal cortex. One survey recorded a 14.5% incidence of hyperplastic nodules, adenomas, and adenocarcinomas. The adrenal cortical lesions are more commonly seen in the males. Neoplasia of the adrenal medulla is rare in hamsters.

Thyroid gland tumors are not commonly diagnosed on gross examination. An incidence of 1.5% to 2.6% has been reported in one colony of hamsters.

Despite the high incidence of adrenal control hyperplasia and adenoma observed in the hamster, clinical disease is rare in the laboratory. Three clinical cases of hyperadrenocorticism have been reported in the long-haired or Teddy Bear hamster [34]. Perhaps this particular strain is more likely to exhibit clinical disease. The animals exhibited the classic signs of Cushing disease (ie, polyuria, polydipsia, polyphagia, alopecia, and hyperpigmentation). One animal responded well to treatment with metyrapone (8 mg by mouth every 24 hours for 30 days), but another was unresponsive to metyrapone at the same dosage and mitotane (5 mg every 24 hours for 30 days). Because there is an increased likelihood that this condition will be seen in private practice, the clinicians should provide more case reports detailing the effectiveness of their treatments in the hamster.

The procedures for adrenalectomy, thyroidectomy, and hypophysectomy are described for the hamster [35]. Because of the likelihood of concurrent disease in geriatric hamsters, the chances for postsurgical survival are low.

The gerbil (*Meriones unguiculatus*)

Other than neoplastic endocrine disease, it is unlikely that a clinician will be confronted with clinical cases of primary endocrine disease in the Mongolian gerbil.

Endocrine anatomy

The gross anatomy and the anatomic location of the endocrine organs are typical of the other rodents. The anatomy has been described elsewhere [36]. Relative to rats and mice, the adrenal glands of the gerbil are large because the gerbil comes from a desert habitat. The kidneys are adept at concentrating the urine to minimize water loss [37], which may be of importance for imaging studies and disease diagnosis.

Diabetes mellitus

Diabetes mellitus has been observed in obese gerbils that were predisposed to hyperglycemia and glucose intolerance [38]. The author suggested that dietary management and gradual weight loss would alleviate the clinical signs.

Because of the presence of only one clinical report in the literature regarding diabetes in the gerbil, it is highly unlikely that the practitioner will be confronted with this clinical entity.

Neoplasia

The reported incidence of neoplasia in the gerbil population older than 2 years of age is 20% [39]. The incidence is greater in the female because of high incidence of neoplasm of the reproductive tract.

The incidence of endocrine tumors is low. The literature only describes tumors in the adrenal cortex (malignant and benign) and an islet cell adenoma of the pancreas. Endocrine neoplasia is not likely to be encountered as a clinical presentation for the practitioner.

Summary

This article summarizes the endocrine diseases of rodents commonly kept as pets. Endocrine disorders are difficult to definitively diagnose but knowledge of these conditions helps the clinician with improved treatment and advanced diagnostic testing options. Information from biomedical research also continues to improve clinical recognition and management of endocrine disease in rodents.

References

[1] Monastersky GM, Geistfeld JG. Transgenic and knockout mice. In: Fox JG, Anderson LC, Lowe FM, et al, editors. Laboratory animal medicine. 2nd edition. San Diego: Academic Press; 2002. p. 1129–41.

[2] Cooper G, Schiller AL. The digestive system. In: Anatomy of the guinea pig. Cambridge: Harvard University Press; 1975. p. 303–24.

[3] Cooper G, Schiller AL. The endocrine system. In: Anatomy of the guinea pig. Cambridge: Harvard University Press; 1975. p. 359–61.

[4] Cooper G, Schiller AL. The central nervous system. In: Anatomy of the guinea pig. Cambridge: Harvard University Press; 1975. p. 235–52.

[5] Hrapkiewiz K, Medina L, Holmes D. Guinea pigs. In: Clinical laboratory animal medicine. 2nd edition. Ames (IA): Blackwell Publishing; 1998. p. 93–116.

[6] O'Rourke D. Disease problems of guinea pigs. In: Queensbury KE, Carpenter JW, editors. Ferrets, rabbits and rodents: clinical medicine and surgery. 2nd edition. Philadelphia: WB Saunders; 2003. p. 245–54.

[7] Feldman EC, Nelson RW. Infertility associated breeding disorders, and disorders of sexual development. In: Canine and feline endocrinology and reproduction. 3rd edition. St. Louis: WB Saunders; 2004. p. 868–900.

[8] Lang CM, Munger BL, Rapp R. Juvenile diabetes mellitus in the guinea pig. In: Andrews EJ, Ward BC, Altman NH, editors. Spontaneous clinical models of humane disease, vol. 1. New York: Academic Press; 1979. p. 139–42.

[9] Flecknell P. Guinea pigs. In: Meredith A, Dednobes S, editors. BSAVA manual of exotic pets. 4th edition. Barcelona: Grafos; 2002. p. 54–64.

[10] Vannevel J. Diabetes mellitus in a 3 year old intact, female guinea pig. Can Vet J 1998;39: 503–4.

[11] Vanneval J. Diabetes in the guinea pig: not uncommon. Can Vet J 1999;40:613.

[12] Johnson-Delaney CA. Small mammal endocrinology. Proc Annu Conf Assoc Avian Vet, Small Mammal and Reptile Program. St. Paul, MN; 1998. p. 99–111.

[13] Manning PJ. Neoplastic disease. In: Wagner JE, Manning PJ, editors. The biology of the guinea pig. New York: Academic Press; 1976. p. 211–25.

[14] Percy DH, Barthold SW. Guinea pigs. In: Pathology of laboratory rodents and rabbits. Ames (IA): Iowa State University Press; 1993. p. 146–78.

[15] Wriston JC Jr, Yellin TO. L-asparaginase: a review. Adv Enzymol 1973;39:185–248.

[16] Debout C. In vitro cytoxic effects of guinea pig natural kill cell (Karloff cells) on homologous leukemia cells (L2C). Leukemia 1993;7:733–5.

[17] Hoar RM. A technique for bilateral adrenalectomy in guinea pigs. Lab Anim Care 1966;16: 410–6.

[18] Hopcroft SC. A technique for the simultaneous bilateral removal of the adrenal glands in guinea pigs, using a new type of safe anesthetic. Exp Med Surg 1966;24:12–9.

[19] Knonka MC, Hoar RM. An improved technique for thyroidectomy in guinea pigs. Lab Anim Sci 1975;25:82–4.

[20] Young WC. Psychobiology of sexual behavior in the guinea pig. Adv Study Behav 1969;2: 1–110.

[21] Hoar RM. Biomethodology. In: Wagner JE, Manning PJ, editors. The biology of the guinea pig. New York: Academic Press; 1976. p. 13–20.

[22] Percy DH, Barthold SW. Guinea pig. In: Pathology of laboratory rodents and rabbits. 2nd edition. Ames (IA): Iowa State University Press; 2001. p. 209–47.

[23] Anver MR, Cohen BJ. Lesions associated with aging. In: Baker HJ, Lindsey JR, Weisbroth SH, editors. The laboratory rat. Biology and disease, vol. I. New York: Academic Press; 1979. p. 378–95.

[24] Popesko P, Rajtova V, Horak J. In: A colour atlas of the anatomy of small laboratory animals, vol. 2. St. Louis: W.B. Saunders; 2002. p. 11–104.

[25] Coleman DL. Diabetes mellitus in rodents. In: Andrews EJ, Ward BC, Altman NH, editors. Spontaneous animal models of human disease, vol. 1. New York: Academic Press; 1979. p. 125–31.

[26] Nakhooda AF, Like AA, Mrliss EB. Diabetes mellitus in the "BB" Wistar rat. In: Andrews EJ, Ward BC, Altman NH, editors. Spontaneous animal models of human disease, vol. 1. New York: Academic Press; 1979. p. 131–6.

[27] Zuchen C, van Sqieten MJ, Solleveld HA, et al. Aging research. In: Foster HL, Small JP, Fox JG, editors. The mouse in biomedical research. vol. IV. Experimental biology and oncology. New York: Academic Press; 1982. p. 11–35.

[28] Coleman DL. Diabetes-obesity syndromes. In: Foster HL, Small JD, Fox JG, editors. The mouse in biomedical research. vol. IV. Experimental biology and oncology. New York: Academic Press; 1982. p. 125–32.

[29] Popesko P, Rajtova V, Horak J. In: A colour atlas of the anatomy of small laboratory animals, vol. 2. St. Louis: W.B. Saunders; 2002. p. 105–66.

[30] Russfield AB. Neoplasms of the endocrine system. In: Foster HL, Small JD, Fox JG, editors. The mouse in biomedical research. vol. IV. Experimental biology and oncology. New York: Acedemic Press; 1982. p. 465–75.

[31] Birwin WS, Olsen GH, Murray KA. Morphophysiology. In: Van Hoosier GL, McPherson CW, editors. Biology of the laboratory hamster. Orlando: Academic Press; 1987. p. 10–41.

[32] Popesko P, Rajtova V, Horak J. In: A colour atlas of the anatomy of small laboratory animals, vol. 2. St. Louis: W.B. Saunders; 2002. p. 167–238.

[33] Robinson FR. Hamster. In: Melby EC, Altman NH, editors. Handbook of laboratory animal science, vol. III. Cleveland: CRC Press; 1976. p. 253–70.

[34] Buck L, Ovr JP, Lawrence KH. Hyperadrenocortism in three teddy bear hamsters. Can Vet J 1984;25:247–50.

[35] Silverman J. Biomethodology. In: Van Hoosier GL, Mc Pherson CW, editors. Biology of the laboratory hamster. Orlando: Academic Press; 1987. p. 70–93.

[36] Williams WW. The anatomy of the Mongolion gerbil (Meriones unquiculates). West Brookfield (MA): Tumblebrook Farm; 1974. p. 1–107.

[37] Percy DH, Barthold SW. Gerbil. In: Pathology of laboratory rodents and rabbits. 2nd edition. Ames (IA): Iowa State University Press; 2001. p. 197–208.

[38] Label-Lard K. Gerbils. In: Handbook of rodent and rabbit medicine. Oxford: Pergaman; 1996. p. 39–58.

[39] Robinson FR. Gerbil. In: Melby EC, Altman NH, editors. Handbook of laboratory animal science, vol. III. Cleveland: CRC Press; 1976. p. 271–3.

ELSEVIER
SAUNDERS

VETERINARY
CLINICS
Exotic Animal Practice

Vet Clin Exot Anim 11 (2008) 163–175

The Reptilian Thyroid and Parathyroid Glands

Sam Rivera, DVM, MS, DABVP–Avian[a],*,
Brad Lock, DVM, DACZM[b]

[a]Department of Animal Health, Zoo Atlanta, 800 Cherokee Avenue SE,
Atlanta, GA 30315-1440, USA
[b]Department of Herpetology, Zoo Atlanta, 800 Cherokee Avenue SE,
Atlanta, GA 30315-1440, USA

The field of reptilian clinical endocrinology is still in its infancy. The thyroid and parathyroid glands are intimately involved with many basic metabolic functions. These glands have been the subject of extensive research studies in reptilian species [1–12]; however, the effects of abnormal gland function have been poorly documented in clinical cases. These glands play a major role in maintaining physiologic homeostasis in all vertebrates. In reptiles, the thyroid gland plays an integral part in ecdysis, reproduction, tail regeneration, growth, endocrine function, and metabolic rate [1–11,13,14]. The parathyroid gland and parathyroid hormone are responsible for maintaining calcium homeostasis. The greatest challenge when attempting to properly document thyroid disease in the clinical setting is the inability to accurately measure hormone levels in the general circulation, particularly at the lower ranges. With the advent of more sensitive assays, however, it should be possible to measure the small amounts of hormones found in reptilian species [15]. The purpose of this article is to review the literature regarding clinical endocrinology of the thyroid and parathyroid glands in reptiles.

Thyroid gland

Anatomy and physiology

The thyroid gland and associated hormones are found in all vertebrate classes. There is minimal variation in the structure of the gland and the

* Corresponding author.
E-mail address: srivera@zooatlanta.org (S. Rivera).

1094-9194/08/$ - see front matter © 2008 Elsevier Inc. All rights reserved.
doi:10.1016/j.cvex.2007.10.002

hormones it produces; however, the hormones have a wide variety of functions. The location and anatomy of the thyroid gland vary among reptile species. In snakes, the thyroid gland is located ventral to the trachea, cranial to the heart base, and caudal to the thymus. It is a single unpaired structure. In lizards and crocodilians, the thyroid gland is located within the ventral cervical region. It may be single, bilobed, or paired, depending on the species [16]. In the green iguana and crocodilians, the paired thyroid glands are joined by a narrow bridge of tissue. In chelonians, the thyroid gland is generally located ventral to the trachea and near the base of the heart. Chelonians have a single unpaired thyroid gland. The tuatara has a single transversely elongate thyroid gland [16].

The functional unit of the thyroid gland is the thyroid follicle. There are numerous follicular acini of varying size lined by squamous or cuboidal epithelium. Each follicle is separated by a single layer of epithelial cells. The follicles are filled with colloid, which is produced by the follicular cells. A capsule surrounds the entire gland, and varying amounts of connective tissue separate the adjacent follicles. The glandular epithelium becomes more cuboidal or columnar during periods of increased thyroid activity and squamous during periods of decreased activity [17]. The follicles show seasonal changes in the dimensions of epithelial cells, extent of enclosed colloid material, presence of desquamated epithelial and blood cells, number of colloid droplets, and varying staining properties of colloid. In soft-shelled turtles, low environmental temperature inhibits thyroid activity and high temperature stimulates the gland activity. It is thought that the environmental temperature acts via the hypothalamo-hypophysial axis, which in turn alters thyroid function in turtles [3,18]. Thyroid hormone levels also vary with season and feeding [19,20]. Thyroid function is mediated centrally via thyrotropin-releasing hormone from the hypothalamus and thyroid-stimulating hormone (TSH) released from the pituitary gland.

Thyroid hormones are important in the growth, development, and metabolism of all vertebrates. In frogs, they are responsible for induction of the many metamorphic changes observed during the postembryonic transition of a tadpole to a juvenile. Thyroid hormones are also important in the molting of reptiles and birds [16]. An interaction between thyroid hormone and reproductive activity has long been recognized in other vertebrates. In birds, it has been proposed that thyroxine (T4) may contribute to seasonal testicular regression by reducing testis sensitivity to LH [21]. Investigations on agamids, lacertids, and geckonids have shown that hypothyroidism induced by thyroidectomy causes a regression of the testis, which involves spermatogenetic arrest and reduction in androgen secretion [22,23]. A thyroid hormone receptor has been found in the testis of lizards (*Podarcis sicula*), which indicates that T3 might be involved in the regulation of gonadal activity. The investigators suggest that in lizards, the combined action of androgens, estrogen, and T3 might regulate testicular activity [24].

Thyroid hormone synthesis is regulated through the hypothalamus-pituitary-thyroid axis, in which thyroid-releasing hormone (or corticotrophin-releasing factor in some species) produced by the hypothalamus stimulates the production of TSH in the pituitary [25,26]. TSH stimulates the production of mainly T4 in the thyroid gland. T4 is transported to peripheral tissues, where it is converted to the more bioactive form 3,3, 5-tri-iodothyronine (T3) through deiodinase activity [25]. T3 functions primarily by regulating gene transcription through high-affinity binding to specific nuclear thyroid hormone receptors that interact with thyroid hormone responsive elements located within the promoters of target genes [27,28]. Blood supply to the thyroid gland is through the left and right thyroid arteries and left and right laryngotracheal arteries, which branch off the external carotids. Venous blood drains from the thyroid vein into the right tracheal vein. The thyroid gland, given its size, receives one of the largest blood supplies of any organ in the body [29].

Thyroid gland functional assessment

Thyroid gland function in mammals is assessed by measuring serum-free and total T4, serum-free and total T3, and serum TSH. Measurement of serum-free thyroxine (fT4) concentration provides a more accurate assessment of thyroid gland function than serum T4 or T3. Techniques for measuring serum fT4 concentration include standard equilibrium dialysis, radioimmunoassay, and a combination of both (modified equilibrium dialysis) [15]. Thyrotropin-releasing hormone and TSH stimulation tests are also used to assess hypothalamo-pituitary-thyroid axis integrity. There are several reports of thyroid assessment in reptiles in which the total T4 was measured; Table 1 lists the reported values [10,15,19,20,30–33]. Tests used to measure thyroid hormones in mammalian species are not sensitive enough to measure the relatively low levels of thyroid hormones found in

Table 1
Reported total T4 values in reptilian species

Species	Total T4 (nmol/L)	Reference
Green iguana (*Iguana iguana*)	3.81 ± 0.84	Hernandez-Divers [30]
Fence lizard (*Sceloporus undulates*)	4.81–6.78	John-Alder [10]
Indian garden lizard (*Calotes versicolor*)	0.21–5.96	Kar [19]
Garter snakes (*Thamnophis sirtalis*)	0.90–1.67	Etheridge [31]
Corn snakes (*Elaphe guttata*)	0.45–6.06	Greenacre [15]
Ball python (*Python regius*)	0.93–4.79	Greenacre [15]
Red-tailed boa (*Boa constrictor*)	≤0.24–3.98	Greenacre [15]
Milk snakes (*Lampropeltis triangulum*)	0.27–2.94	Greenacre [15]
Common cobra (*Naja naja*)	12.87–25.74	Wong [32]
Desert tortoise (*Gopherus agassizii*)	0.35–4	Kohel [20]
Eastern snake-necked turtle (*Chelodina longicollis*)	0.69 ± 0.11	Hulbert [5]

reptilian blood. The lack of validated thyroid function tests for reptilian species has slowed progress in this area. Recently, a method for using high-sensitivity radioimmunoassay to measure total T4 in snakes was reported [15].

Diseases affecting the thyroid gland

Thyroid gland dysfunction is poorly documented in reptiles. Thyroid dysfunction can be caused by improper light cycles, improper hibernation, and improper thermal gradients. As with many conditions in reptiles, husbandry management must be taken into account when assessing thyroid gland function. Some of the conditions affecting the thyroid gland of reptiles that have been reported include goiter secondary to iodine deficiency or toxicity, hyperthyroidism, hypothyroidism, and neoplasia. However, the prevalence of thyroid disease in reptiles resulting in metabolic derangements is unknown.

Iodine deficiency

The thyroid gland is the only tissue in the body able to accumulate a large amount of iodine and incorporate it into hormones. The metabolism of iodine is closely related to thyroid function. Dietary iodine, an essential trace mineral, is absorbed in the small intestine and plays an essential role in metabolism as a component of thyroid hormones. Deficiency of iodine has been associated with stillbirths, abortion, prolonged gestation, congenital malformations, mental retardation, dwarfism, stunted growth, skin problems, decreased metabolic rate, and increased mortality in mammals. In reptiles, the most common clinical sign is goiter, an enlargement of the thyroid gland. Iodine deficiency leads to decreased blood hormone levels, which activates the hypothalamo-pituitary axis leading to increased TSH production and resulting in hypertrophy and hyperplasia of the thyroid follicular cells. Goiter has been reported in tortoises and reportedly is more prevalent in giant tortoises from the Galapagos and Aldabra Islands [33,34].

Anything that affects the availability of iodine may induce goiter. Herbivorous reptiles fed diets grown in iodine-deficient soils, which occur worldwide, can be affected. Another important cause includes dietary goitrogens, which are found in bok choy, broccoli, cabbage, cauliflower, kale, mustard seed, rapeseed, soy bean sprouts, and turnips. The effects of these food items can be exacerbated if an animal is fed a marginal iodine-deficient diet. These food items should be fed intermittently and should not comprise a large percent of the herbivorous reptile diet. Since the development of formulated diets for herbivorous reptiles and increased public awareness of reptilian dietary needs, the incidence of goiter caused by iodine deficiency has decreased significantly. However, it must be at the top of the differential list for any reptile that presents with thyroid gland enlargement [35].

Iodine toxicity

This condition presents as goiter because of the impaired iodine use. The most common cause is oversupplementation of iodine in the diet [35]. Elevated blood iodine levels interfere with thyroxinogenesis, which leads to lowered blood thyroid levels. Excess iodine also seems to block the release of T3 and T4 from the follicles by interfering with proteolysis of colloid by lysosomes [36].

Hyperthyroidism

Hyperthyroidism is defined as a pathologic and sustained state of high metabolism caused by an elevated concentration of thyroid hormones in the circulation. In mammals, hyperthyroidism leads to chronic cellular malnutrition, decreased gastrointestinal transit time, malabsorption, hepatocellular damage, myocardial hypertrophy, hypertension, and increased glomerular filtration rate [36]. Causes of hyperthyroidism include hyperfunctioning thyroid nodules, thyroid neoplasia, oversupplementation of exogenous thyroid hormone, and pituitary dysfunction leading to increased TSH secretion, which results in increased T4 production. There is one report of hyperthyroidism in a green iguana that resembled feline hyperthyroidism [30]. The presenting clinical signs included weight loss, polyphagia, hyperactivity, increased aggression, loss of dorsal spines, and tachycardia. The diagnosis was based on an elevated T4 level (30 nmol/L), which was significantly higher than the level measured in clinically healthy adult iguanas (3.81 $\pm$ 0.84 nmol/L). The animal had a palpable bilobed mass in the ventral cervical region near the thoracic inlet. The increased T4 level was caused by a functional thyroid follicular adenoma. Thyroidectomy was curative. The blood T4 was at the level of clinically healthy adults 173 days after surgery.

Hyperthyroidism has been suspected in snakes that undergo frequent ecdysis. It was suspected in an older corn snake (*Elaphe guttata*) that shed its skin every 2 weeks. The snake responded to methimazole (1 mg/kg/d) by returning to a more regular ecdysis cycle [17]. The diagnosis of hyperparathyroidism in these cases was based on response to therapy and not blood hormone levels. The diagnosis of hyperthyroidism is characterized by an elevated T4 level and accompanying clinical signs. Current laboratory assays are able to measure reptilian T4; however, validated assays to test samples from many reptilian species have not been reported. The two hyperthyroidism treatment modalities that have been reported in reptiles are thyroidectomy and antithyroid drugs [17,30]. Radioactive therapy is safe and effective in treating feline hyperthyroidism, but its use has not been reported in reptiles.

Hypothyroidism

Hypothyroidism is characterized by decreased production and release of thyroid hormones resulting in decreased metabolic activity. This condition has been documented in reptiles [17,33,34]. Hypothyroidism in chelonians fed goitrogenic diets has been described based on clinical and histopathologic evaluations; however, thyroid function was not assessed by laboratory methods [17,34]. Clinical signs of hypothyroidism in reptiles include decreased appetite, lethargy, depression, obesity, dysecdysis, stunting, myxedema, and goiter. The most commonly reported causes of hypothyroidism in reptiles are associated with conditions that interfere with normal thyroid function, such as iodine deficiency or toxicity and feeding excessive amounts of goitrogenic food items. Bilateral thyroidectomy can lead to hypothyroidism. Hernandez-Divers and colleagues [30] did not observe evidence of hypothyroidism in an iguana that underwent thyroidectomy for the treatment of hyperthyroidism associated with a functional thyroid adenoma. The iguana was euthyroid 173 days after surgery. Reptiles, like many mammals, have accessory thyroid tissues that can become hyperplastic and produce thyroid hormones.

The diagnosis of hypothyroidism in mammals is based on measuring T4 levels in the general circulation. Subnormal T4 levels are suggestive of but not diagnostic for hypothyroidism. High TSH levels with low T4 concentration are indicative of hypothyroidism. The TSH stimulation test is the gold standard in mammals for the diagnosis of hypothyroidism; however, this test has not been validated in reptilian species. The diagnosis of hypothyroidism in reptiles using laboratory methods to measure thyroid hormones and TSH has not been well documented largely because of the absence of validated assays in reptilian species.

Neoplasia

Thyroid neoplasia reports in reptiles are common [17,30,37–43]. Thyroid adenomas or carcinomas have been reported in lizards [30,36,38,39], snakes [40], and several chelonian species [41]. Some of the species affected include *Iguana iguana*, *Cordylus polyzonus*, *Varanus komodoensis*, *Chrysemys picta*, and *Varanus salvator*. Most of the cases were incidental findings during necropsy, and it is not known what the thyroid hormone status was in the general circulation before death. In one case, thyroidectomy was successful in the treatment of a functional thyroid adenoma that had resulted in hyperthyroidism in a green iguana [30].

Endocrine-disrupting contaminants

Recent studies have documented abnormal thyroid activity in reptiles as a result of exposure to environmental chemicals [44]. These chemicals are known as endocrine-disrupting contaminants. Thyroid gland disruption as a result of endocrine-disrupting contaminant exposure has been well documented in several vertebrate classes [45,46]. Increased blood T4 and decreased T3 levels were seen in freshwater catfish (*Clarias batrachus*) exposed to endosulfan (an organochlorine pesticide), which suggests that this pesticide blocks extrathyroidal conversion of T4 to T3 [47]. Carbaryl caused a decrease in T4 levels and an increase in T3 levels in *C batrachus* [47]. Hypothyroidism in weanling male rats was induced by administration of the polychlorinated biphenyl (PCB) mixture Aroclor 1254 [48]. Several studies have documented structural abnormalities in the thyroid glands of wildlife exposed to endocrine-disrupting contaminants. Abnormally large follicles with cuboidal or squamous epithelium and depleted colloid have been observed in herring gulls from the Great Lakes basin, an area where thyroid disorders, characterized by structural abnormalities, have been documented in fish, avian, and mammal species [49,50]. These structural abnormalities are suspected to have an environmental cause [51]. Thyroid gland abnormalities have been noted in American alligators (*Alligator mississippiensis*), a species highly susceptible to endocrine disruption by contamination [52]. Abnormalities associated with endocrine-disrupting contaminants exposure in juvenile alligators include altered sex-steroid concentrations, abnormal thyroid hormone blood levels, altered gonadal morphology, and reduced phallus size [53]. Exposure to environmental contaminants must be taken into account when assessing overall thyroid disruptions in reptiles.

Parathyroid gland

Anatomy and physiology

The parathyroid glands are present in all air-breathing vertebrates; one or two pairs are present. In most mammals, one or both parathyroid gland pairs are closely associated with the thyroid gland. In reptiles, the glands are separated from the thyroid gland [54]. The location of the parathyroid gland varies among different reptilian species; generally the anterior pair is associated with the carotid artery and the posterior pair is associated with the aortic arch. In snakes, the anterior pair is associated with the carotid artery near the mandibular ramus [12]. Lizards may have one or two pairs of parathyroid gland. In green iguanas, the anterior parathyroid glands are located along the medial surface of the mandibular rami, and the posterior pair is located at the origins of the internal and external carotid arteries. Chelonians have two pairs of parathyroid glands. The anterior pair is located within the thymus, and the posterior pair is caudal to the aortic arch and cranial to the heart. Crocodilians may have one or two pairs of parathyroid glands located near the common carotid artery [12]. The parenchyma of the parathyroid gland in reptiles consists largely of chief cells, which are arranged in cords separated by connective tissue that contains a capillary network [12,55]. The chief cells are involved in the production and release of parathyroid hormone (PTH). The oxyphil cells present is some vertebrates are not found in the parathyroid gland of most reptile species [55].

The primary hormones involved in calcium homeostasis are the parathyroid hormone, calcitonin, and vitamin D3. A detailed discussion of calcium metabolism in reptiles is beyond the scope of this article. The reader is referred to Campbell [56] and Mader [57] for a review of calcium metabolism in reptiles. The parathyroid hormone is responsible for maintaining normal blood calcium concentration. The total calcium in the general circulation is composed of two fractions: protein bound and diffusible fraction (ionized calcium). The biologically active form of calcium (ionized) plays a major role in many biologic processes, including muscle contractions, blood coagulation, enzyme activity, neural excitability, hormone release, and membrane permeability. The control of ionized calcium is vital for normal function in all vertebrates. The sites of PTH action are the bones, kidneys, intestines, endolymphatics, and dermal skeleton; however, these actions have not been well investigated in reptiles [12]. Low levels of ionized calcium in the blood stimulate the release of PTH, which results in calcium resorption from the bones, increased calcium resorption from the kidneys, and increased calcium absorption from the intestines. Increased ionized calcium in the general circulation has a negative effect on the release of PTH. It has been suggested that in some turtle species PTH is not the main factor for the regulation of calcium homeostasis [12].

Diseases of the parathyroid gland

Primary parathyroid disorders have not been well documented in reptiles. The most common conditions that lead to parathyroid gland disorders in reptiles are inadequate calcium or vitamin D3 supplementation leading to nutritional secondary hyperparathyroidism or severe chronic renal disease causing a disturbance in the metabolism of vitamin D3 and calcium and phosphorous homeostasis leading to renal secondary hyperparathyroidism [57]. Hyperparathyroidism is a metabolic disorder in which excessive amounts of PTH secreted by the parathyroid glands cause disturbances of calcium homeostasis (Fig. 1).

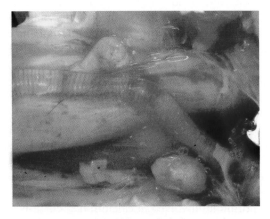

Fig. 1. Parathyroid hyperplasia in a tortoise.

Nutritional secondary hyperparathyroidism

Nutritional secondary hyperparathyroidism (NSHP) often occurs as a result of inadequate diet or inappropriate husbandry. This condition is characterized by an increase in the production of PTH by the parathyroid gland in response to hypocalcemia [58]. This increase leads to increased calcium resorption from the bones, which leads to osteopenia and weak bones. Juvenile reptiles with NSHP commonly have metabolic bone disease manifested as fibrous osteodystrophy and pathologic fractures. Common predisposing factors for the development of NSHP include decrease dietary calcium, vitamin D3 deficiency, improper calcium/phosphorous ratio, and inadequate exposure to ultraviolet radiation in diurnal species. In chelonians, NSHP may predispose the animal to hepatic lipidosis, soft shell, carapacial deformities, and renal disease [59]. In mammals, PTH has been shown to adversely affect lipid metabolism [60]. PTH is also a powerful modulator of renal blood flow and glomerular filtration rate [61]. Excessive PTH seems to be nephrotoxic [62]. Common clinical signs associated with NSHP include thickening and swelling of the long bones and mandible, pathologic fractures of long bones and spine, horizontal rotation of the scapula, tetany, muscle fasciculation, hyperreflexia, cloacal or rectal prolapse, anorexia, and stunted growth [57].

Initial therapy should address presenting complaints, such as fractures and life-threatening hypocalcemia. Many cases require oral calcium supplementations for months before recovery is complete. Initial supplementation of parenteral vitamin D3 once weekly for 2 weeks has proved useful [63]. Calcitonin administration has been used in the treatment of NSHP in green iguanas [64]. It must be done carefully, however, because administration of calcitonin to hypocalcemic patients can be fatal. The main objective of long-term treatment, once a patient is stable, is to correct the underlying predisposing factors that led to the development of NSHP. One must keep in mind that other factors yet unknown may predispose reptiles to this condition.

Renal secondary hyperparathyroidism

Renal secondary hyperparathyroidism is a condition that is a consequence of chronic renal failure. Impaired renal function leads to hyperphosphatemia. As the concentration of phosphorus increases, blood calcium levels decrease. Hypocalcemia is further aggravated by a disruption of vitamin D3 metabolism in the failing renal tissue, which results in decreased calcium absorption from the intestines. The end result is hypocalcemia, which leads to hyperparathyroidism. The goal of treatment is to correct the primary renal disease [57].

Neoplasia

Parathyroid neoplasia has been reported in reptiles. A parathyroid adenoma was described in a red footed tortoise (*Geochelone carbonaria*). The tortoise had clinical signs consistent with hyperparathyroidism (soft and deformed carapace and plastron). The animal was euthanized, and the diagnosis of primary hyperparathyroidism caused by a parathyroid adenoma was confirmed via histopathology [65].

Summary

The clinical endocrinology referable to the thyroid and parathyroid glands of reptiles is in its infancy, whereas the anatomy and location of these glands between orders of reptiles is better known. These two glands are involved in the regulation and mediation of several physiologic processes in reptiles, including shedding cycles, reproduction, growth, and changes in metabolic rate. However, few published reports of normal reference ranges for thyroid and parathyroid hormone plasma concentrations have been published. The limited reported values in reptiles suggest that variability exists in the concentration of these hormones between orders, species, and individuals.

Although a few diseases and disorders of the thyroid and parathyroid glands in reptiles are clinically well described, such as NSHP, renal secondary hyperparathyroidism, and goiter, other well-known disorders seen in mammals, including iodine toxicity, hyperthyroidism, hypothyroidism, neoplasia, and environmental contaminant effects on the glands, are poorly documented. However, the few published reports describing some of these disorders suggest a clinical similarity in these diseases between reptiles and mammals. Given the wide range of physiologic functions that these glands and associated hormones regulate and moderate, clinical disorders and disease secondary to thyroid and parathyroid dysfunction in reptiles are probably underdiagnosed. This situation will improve as hormonal assays become more widely available, additional case reports and controlled studies are published, and the understanding of clinical disorders of the thyroid and parathyroid glands in reptiles increases.

References

[1] Al-Sadoon MK, el-Banna AA. The effects of thyroxine on the oxygen consumption of the ocellated skink, *Chalcides ocellatus*. Comp Biochem Physiol A 1987;86:189–92.

[2] Chandola-Saklani A, Kar A. Evidence of the role of thyroxine as a hormone in the physiology of the lizard. Gen Comp Endocrinol 1990;78:173–9.

[3] Chui KW, Sham JS, Maderson PF, et al. Interaction between thermal environments and hormones affecting skin-shedding frequency in the tokay (*Gekko gecko*). Comp Biochem Physiol A 1986;84:345–51.

[4] Gerwien RW, John-Alder HB. Growth and behavior of thyroid deficient lizards (*Sceloporus undulatus*). Gen Comp Endocrinol 1992;87:312–24.

[5] Hulbert AJ, Williams CA. Thyroid function in a lizard, a tortoise and a crocodile, compared with mammals. Comp Biochem Physiol A 1988;90:41–8.

[6] Jacob V, Oommen OV. Intermediary metabolism in a lizard, *Calotes versicolor*: role of thyroid hormones. Gen Comp Endocrinol 1990;77:324–6.

[7] John-Alder HB. Effects of thyroxine supplementation on metabolic rate and aerobic capacity in a lizard. Am J Physiol 1983;244:659–66.

[8] John-Alder HB. Reduced aerobic capacity and locomotory endurance in thyroid-deficient lizards. J Exp Biol 1984;109:175–89.

[9] John-Alder HB. Thyroid regulation of resting metabolic rate and intermediary metabolic enzymes in a lizard (*Sceloporus occidentalis*). Gen Comp Endocrinol 1990;77:56–62.

[10] John-Alder HB, Joos B. Interactive effects of thyroxine and experimental location on running endurance, tissue masses, and enzyme activities in captive versus field-active lizards (*Sceloporus undulatus*). Gen Comp Endocrinol 1991;81:120–32.

[11] Ramachandran AV, Swamy MS, Kurup AK. Local and systemic alterations in cyclic 3′,5′AMP phosphodiesterase activity in relation to tail regeneration under hypothyroidism and T4 replacement in the lizard, *Mabuya carinata*. Mol Reprod Dev 1996;45:48–51.

[12] Srivastav AK, Sasayama Y, Suzuki N. Morphology and physiological significance of parathyroid glands in reptilia. Microsc Res Tech 1995;32(2):91–103.

[13] Gans C, Parsons TS. Morphology. In: Gans C, Gaunt AS, editors. Biology of the reptilia. New York: Academic Press; 1970.

[14] Hulbert AJ, Else PL. Comparison of the "mammal machine" and the "reptile machine": energy use and thyroid activity. Am J Physiol 1981;241:350–6.

[15] Greenacre CB, Young DW, Behrend EN, et al. Validation of a novel high-sensitivity radioimmunoassay procedure for measurement of total thyroxine concentration in psittacine birds and snakes. Am J Vet Res 2001;62(11):1750–4.

[16] Lynn WG. The thyroid. In: Gans C, Parson TS, editors. Biology of reptilia. New York: Academic Press; 1970. p. 201–34.

[17] Frye FL. Biomedical and surgical aspects of captive reptile husbandry. 2nd edition. FL: Krieger Publishing; 1991.

[18] Sengupta BA, Ray PP, Chaudhuri-Sengupta S, et al. Thyroidal modulation following hypo- and hyperthermia in the soft-shelled turtle *Lissemys punctata punctata*. Eur J Morphol 2003; 41(5):149–54.

[19] Kar A, Chandola-Saklani A. Circulating thyroid hormone concentrations in relation to seasonal events in the male Indian garden lizard, *Calotes versicolor*. Gen Comp Endocrinol 1985;60:14–9.

[20] Kohel KA, MacKenzie DS, Rostal DC, et al. Seasonality in plasma thyroxine in the desert tortoise, *Gopherus agassizii*. Gen Comp Endocrinol 2001;121:214–22.

[21] Jallageas M, Follet BK, Assenmacher I. Thyroid-gonadal interactions during the postnuptial phase of the sexual cycle in male ducks. Gen Comp Endocrinol 1978;34:68–9.

[22] Plowman MM, Lynn WG. The role of the thyroid in testicular function in the gecko, *Cleonyx variegates*. Gen Comp Endocrinol 1973;20:342–6.

[23] Haldar-Misra CM, Thapliyal JP. Thyroid in reproduction in reptiles. Gen Comp Endocrinol 1981;43:537–42.

[24] Cardone A, Angelini F, Esposito T, et al. The expression of androgen receptor messenger RNA is regulated by tri-iodothyronine in lizard testis. J Steroid Biochem Mol Biol 2000;72:133–41.

[25] Norris DO. Vertebrate endocrinology. San Diego: Academic Press; 1997.

[26] Denver R. Evolution of the corticotropin-releasing hormone signaling system and its role in stress-induced phenotypic plasticity. Ann N Y Acad Sci 1999;897:46–53.

[27] Bassett J, Harvey CB, Williams GR. Mechanisms of thyroid hormone receptor-specific nuclear and extra nuclear actions. Mol Cell Endocrinol 2003;213:1–11.

[28] Helbing CC, Crump K, Bailey CM, et al. Isolation of the alligator (*Alligator mississippiensis*) thyroid hormone receptor and transcripts and their responsiveness to thyroid stimulating hormone. Gen Comp Endocrinol 2006;149:141–50.

[29] Oldham JC, Smith HM. Laboratory anatomy of the green iguana. Dubuque (IA): W.M.C. Brown; 1975.

[30] Hernandez-Divers SJ, Knott CD, MacDonald J. Diagnosis and surgical treatment of thyroid adenoma-induced hyperthyroidism in a green iguana (*Iguana iguana*). J Zoo Wildl Med 2001;32(4):465–75.

[31] Etheridge K. Thyroxine-induced changes in metabolic rate and cytochrome oxidase activity in *Thamnophis sirtalis*: effects of nutritional status. Gen Comp Endocrinol 1993;91:66–73.

[32] Wong KL, Chiu KW, Wong CC. The snake thyroid gland: I. Seasonal variation of thyroidal and serum iodoamino acids. Gen Comp Endocrinol 1974;23:63–70.

[33] Norton TM, Jacobson RE, Caligiuri R, et al. Medical management of a Galapagos tortoise (*Geochelone elephantopus*) with hypothyroidism. J Zoo Wildl Med 1989;20:212–6.

[34] Frye FL, Dutra FR. Hypothyroidism in turtles and tortoises. Vet Med Small Anim Clin 1974;69:990–3.

[35] Donoghue S. Nutrition. In: Mader DR, editor. Reptile medicine and surgery. 2nd edition. St. Louis, MO: Elsevier Inc.; 2006. p. 251–98.

[36] Capen CC, Martin SL. The thyroid gland. In: McDonald LE, Pineda MH, editors. Veterinary endocrinology and reproduction. 4th edition. Philadelphia: Lea & Febiger; 1989. p. 58–91.

[37] Harshbarger JC. Activities report registry of tumors in lower animals, 1965–1973. Washington, DC: Smithsonian Institute; 1974.

[38] Harshbarger JC. Activities report registry of tumors in lower animals, 1975 supplement. Washington, DC: Smithsonian Institute; 1975.

[39] Whiteside DP, Garner MM. Thyroid adenocarcinoma in a crocodile lizard, *Shinisaurus crocodilurus*. J Herp Med Surg 2001;11:13–6.

[40] Ramsay EC, Munson L, Lowestein L, et al. A retrospective study of neoplasia in a collection of captive snakes. J Zoo Wildl Med 1996;27(1):28–34.

[41] Machotka SV. Neoplasia in reptiles. In: Hoff GL, Frye FL, Jacobson ER, editors. Diseases of amphibians and reptiles. New York: Plenum Press; 1984. p. 519–80.

[42] Cowan DF. Diseases of captive reptiles. J Am Vet Med Assoc 1968;153(7):848–59.

[43] Garner MM, Hernandez-Divers SM, Raymond JT. Reptile neoplasia: a retrospective study of case submissions to a specialty diagnostic service. Vet Clin North Am Exot Anim Pract 2004;7(3):653–71.

[44] Hewitt EA, Crain DA, Gunderson MP, et al. Thyroid status in juvenile alligators (*Alligator mississippiensis*) from contaminated and reference sites on Lake Okeechobee, Florida, USA. Chemosphere 2002;47:1129–35.

[45] Leatherland JF. Endocrine and reproductive function in Great Lakes salmon. In: Colborn T, Clement C, editors. Chemically-induced alterations in sexual and functional development: the wildlife/human connection. Princeton (MN): Princeton Scientific; 1992. p. 129–46.

[46] Leatherland JF. Contaminant-altered thyroid function in wildlife. In: Guillette LJ, Crain DA, editors. Environmental endocrine disruptors: an evolutionary perspective. New York: Taylor and Francis; 2000. p. 155–81.

[47] Sinha N, Lal B, Singh TP. Pesticides induced changes in circulating thyroid hormones in the freshwater catfish (*Clarias batrachus*). Comp Biochem Physiol A 1991;100:107–10.

[48] Gray LE, Ostby J, Marshall R, et al. Reproductive and thyroid effects of low-level polychlorinated biphenyl (Aroclor 1254) exposure. Fundam Appl Toxicol 1993;20:288–94.

[49] Moccia RD, Fox GA, Britton A. A quantitative assessment of thyroid histopathology of herring gulls (*Larus argentatus*) from the Great Lakes and a hypothesis on the causal role of environmental contaminants. J Wildl Dis 1986;22:60–70.

[50] Leatherland JF. Reflections on the thyroidology of fishes: from molecules to humankind. Guelph Ichthyol Rev 1994;2:1–67.

[51] Moccia RD, Leatherland JF, Sonstegard RA. Quantitative interlake comparison of thyroid pathology in Great Lakes coho (*Oncorhynchus kisutch*) and Chinook (*Oncorhynchus tschawytscha*) salmon. Cancer Res 1981;41:2200–10.

[52] Crain DA, Guillette LJ. Reptiles as models of contaminant-induced endocrine disruption. Anim Reprod Sci 1998;53:77–86.

[53] Crain DA, Guillette LJ, Pickford DB, et al. Sex-steroid and thyroid hormone concentrations in juvenile alligators (*Alligator mississippiensis*) from contaminated and reference lakes in Florida, USA. Environ Toxicol Chem 1998;17:446–52.

[54] Shoumura S, Emura S, Isono H. The parathyroid gland under normal and experimental conditions. Kaibogaku Zasshi 1993;68(1):5–29.

[55] Yoshidaterasawa K, Hayakawa D, Chen H, et al. Fine structure of the parathyroid gland of the snake, *Elaphe quadrivirgata*. Okajimas Folia Anat Jpn 1998;75(2–3):141–53.

[56] Campbell TW. Clinical pathology of reptiles. In: Mader DR, editor. Reptile medicine and surgery. 2nd edition. St. Louis (MO): Elsevier Inc.; 2006. p. 453–79.

[57] Mader DR. Metabolic bone disease. In: Mader DR, editor. Reptile medicine and surgery. 2nd edition. St. Louis (MO): Elsevier Inc.; 2006. p. 841–51.

[58] Capen CC. The calcium regulating hormones: parathyroid hormone, calcitonin, and cholecalciferol. In: McDonald LE, Pineda MH, editors. Veterinary endocrinology and reproduction. 4th edition. Philadelphia: Lea & Febiger; 1989. p. 92–185.

[59] McArthur S, Meyer J, Innis C. Anatomy and physiology. In: McArthur S, Wilkinson R, Meyer J, editors. Medicine and surgery of tortoises and turtles. Oxford (NY): Blackwell publishing Ltd.; 2004. p. 35–72.

[60] Akmal M, Kasim SE, Soliman AR, et al. Excess parathyroid hormone adversely affects lipid metabolism in chronic renal failure. Kidney Int 1990;37(3):854–8.

[61] Massfelder T, Parekh N, Endlich K, et al. Effect of intrarenally infused parathyroid hormone-related protein on renal blood flow and glomerular filtration rate in the anaesthetized rat. Br J Pharmacol 1996;118(8):1995–2000.

[62] Rosol TJ, Chew DJ, Nagode LA, et al. Pathophysiology of calcium metabolism. Vet Clin Pathol 1995;24(2):49–63.

[63] Boyer TH. Metabolic bone disease. In: Mader DR, editor. Reptile medicine and surgery. Philadelphia: WB Saunders; 1996. p. 385–92.

[64] Mader DR. Use of calcitonin in green iguanas (*Iguana iguana*) with metabolic bone disease. Bull Assoc Reptil Amphib Vet 1993;3(1):5.

[65] Frye FL, Carney JD. Parathyroid adenoma in a tortoise. Vet Med Small Anim Clin 1975; 70(5):582–4.

ELSEVIER
SAUNDERS

VETERINARY
CLINICS
Exotic Animal Practice

Vet Clin Exot Anim 11 (2008) 177–194

Index

Note: Page numbers of article titles are in **boldface** type.

Moving?

Make sure your subscription moves with you!

To notify us of your new address, find your **Clinics Account Number** (located on your mailing label above your name), and contact customer service at:

E-mail: elspcs@elsevier.com

800-654-2452 (subscribers in the U.S. & Canada)
407-345-4000 (subscribers outside of the U.S. & Canada)

Fax number: 407-363-9661

Elsevier Periodicals Customer Service
6277 Sea Harbor Drive
Orlando, FL 32887-4800

*To ensure uninterrupted delivery of your subscription, please notify us at least 4 weeks in advance of move.